GLIMPSES OF INDIAN VETERINARY SCIENCE

GLIMPSES OF INDIAN VETERINARY SCIENCE

Dr. Rishendra Verma
B.Sc., BVSc.&AH, MVSc (Bact), M.Sc.(Immunol, UK)
Ph.D(Bact), Dip. Journalism (Mysore)

2018
Daya Publishing House®
A Division of
Astral International Pvt. Ltd.
New Delhi - 110 002

First Published, 2000
Reprinted, 2018

ISBN: 978-81-7035-224-2 (Hardbound)

Published by : **Daya Publishing House®**
A Division of
Astral International Pvt. Ltd.
– ISO 9001:2008 Certified Company –
4736/23, Ansari Road, Darya Ganj
New Delhi-110 002
Ph. 011-43549197, 23278134
E-mail: info@astralint.com
Website: www.astralint.com

PREFACE

Veterinary Science flourished in ancient India and persons serving as animal doctors have existed since earliest times. Veterinary science as it is viewed today has developed through several stages. I remember that during my studentship at Mathura I wrote an article entitled "Veterinary and Veterinarians". My idea of writing on these lines lingered on and an article entitled "Veterinary Science and Journalism in India" could be published in 1992 in the souvenir of Indian Association for the Advancement of Veterinary Research, Bareilly. My thinking was further strengthened by publication "Glimpses of Veterinary Profession (1991)" by Dr. Y. T. Gadre; Review of Animal Science Journalism in India by R.R. Lokeshwar in 1994. I also wrote a paper "Veterinary Research in India-Present, Past and Future for its inclusion in the book entitiled "Educational Research in India" to be published by Dr. S. P. Ahluwalia,Institute of National and Foreign Languages, Bhilai (MP). Time to time interaction on the subject of veterinary science and journals with concerned persons and the above background encouraged me to take up this fascinating assignment of writing the present book. In fact, there is no such publication which would provide information on various aspects of development of veterinary science and its other activities. The present write up is indeed a `Mirror of the Esteemed Veterinary Science in India'. It provides good informations on the past, present and most profound progress of veterinary science. This book will certainly be harbinger for our readers because the publication of this book has been brought through thick and thin.

The book has been divided into several sections and right from the Etmyology of "Veterinary", the book contains materials on Veterinary Science, International Organisations, National

Bodies, Academies, Research Institutes, Universities, Veterinary Colleges, Journals and Periodicals, Professional Societies, Awards, Information Systems and Important Publications. It was really a herculian task to gather data on such varying aspects and probably with the cooperation of Dean, Veterinary Colleges, Secretaries and editors of many associations, Directors of various Institutes, Dr. Rama Kumar, V, Secretary, Veterinary Council of India, it could be possible to present this book.

The book would serve as a 'torch bearer' to those who wish to know about veterinary science, education, research and veterinary profession. Although, much care has been taken , the possibility of omissions can not be ruled out. It is hoped that this publication would be much appreciated.

Rishendra Verma

CONTENTS

Chapter - 1

The Etymology of "Veterinary"

Fussing over the etymology of "veterinary", "veterinarian", "veterinary surgeon", "veterinaire", "veterinara" etc as employed in the Latin and Anglo-Saxon tongues, is probably expected of a writer of veterinary history. The word is just a pleonastic freak that has crept into these languages without invitation, lasting welcome, or hope of departure. The fault is that it has no medical siginificance and certainly no medical origin. The word "veterinary" [L veterinarius, Fr.veterinare] is the Latin adjective "veterinus" and never had a noun form until "veterinarian" somewhere and somehow was coined. Verrius Flaccus (14 AD) a grammarian gives the verb form as *vebere* to draw, and defines the term "veterinarinus" as " any animal that works with a yoke" or "pertaining to beasts of burden". Veterinarian is one who practice veterinary medicine and surgery. In other words a veterinarian has been defined as one skilled in or treating diseases, injuries of animals; a doctor of veterinary medicine.

Chapter - 2

Blue Cross

The Encyclopaedia Brittanica refers only to this non-profit organisation which pays hospital expenses. Webster's International Dictionary of the English Languauge, 1933 edition under New Words states:

"Blue Cross (a) A branch founded in 1912 by an English Society, "Our Dumb Friends' League" for the succor of horses and dogs. It was active in the Balkan Wars (912-13) and the World war (b) A Society [American Blue Cross Society] formed in the United States in 1914 for the humane treatment of animals".

The British Government in the First World War conferred a function on the Royal SPCA to operate as an auxillary i.e., Blue Cross, to the Royal Army Veterinary Corps in 1914. In fact, its personnel and other materials were used in the European theatres of The Ailied Powers which did not include the United States. " ...... At the 52nd Annual Meetings of the American Veterinary Medical Association in Oakland, California, in 1915, the blue crosses adorned the menu at the banquet and the front cover page of the convention programme. They were worn in the form of lapel buttons by the conventioners. At the next year's meeting, a special committee on the Emblem chaired by D. M. Campbell reported adoption of the "Blue Cross" as an insignia for this association, the cross retained same shape and of the same dimensions as the Clara Barton Cross (Clara Barton, founder, Red Cross) either plain or set in gray or white circular background". In 1915, a Chicago sales company advertised the availability of a blue cross enamelled emblem (4.5" diameter) which could be attached to veterinarians automobiles or buggies; a blue cross lapel button also was advertised".

The above description has been taken from a History of Blue Cross, by Dr. Kenneth. B. Hass published in the Indian Veterinary Journal, Vol. 19: 1995 with courtesy of Dr. G. S. Khatra, Editor, Punjab Veterinarian.

In India, it could not be known from published literature as to when the Blue cross was adopted, however, it appears that Blue Cross insignia has been in use since long time.

Societies have been created e.g., `International Blue Cross Organisation" in 1986, C-171, Sector, C, Mahanagar, Lucknow. However, there is no agile Blue Cross Society as such except for fact that the Blue Cross is used universally in veterinary science in various types of emblems in India.

Chapter - 3

VETERINARY SCIENCE

"India was veritably an apotheosis of the animal world and even the most irreverent layman would see (in ancient Indian Medical and Veterinary Literature), the distinct forerunner of all the scientific and surgical marvels of today"- **Recorded by Johnston Saint of Historical Museum, London.**

Ancient India

Veterinary science flourished in ancient India, where separate treaties on the diseases of horses and elephants were written, and there were hospitals for various species of animals. The legal code of the Babylonian king Hammurabi (c,1800 B.C.) prescribed the fees for "doctors of asses and oxen", and the Egyptian papyrus of Kahun (1900 B.C.) revealed that prescriptions were given for diseases in dogs and cattle. The ancient Greeks had a class of *hippiatori* (literally, "horse doctor") and a number of writers (Hippocrates, b 460 B.C. ; Aristotle, b, 384 B. C.) gave consideration to the treatment of animal diseases. Indian scientific works were mostly written in Sanskrit, being the cultural language in 500 B. C. There was considerable interchange of scientific informations with the Arabs from the seventh century AD. Indian science as such remained unknown in Europe until the end of eighteenth century. Specialization in veterinary science has been realized in epics (1000 B. C) with three major heads comprising horses, cattle and elephants. The history of veterinary science in ancient times can be traced up to the Post-Vedic period. Palakapya, the well known ancient surgeon wrote, on the art of breeding and treating elephants. Kautalaya has described in his Arthasastra establishment of an organised livestock department under

Chandragupta Maurya (322-298 BC). It is also evident from the perusal of literature that Ashoka founded hospitals and dispensaries for men and animals throughout the Kingdom. In the "SHUKRAN III" of ninth century, it is written that the superintendent of State departments for each variety of domesticated animals needed special qualification in veterinary subjects and after him the veterinary science was known as Salihotra or Saluteri. In Mongal regime, Ain-1-Akbari contained good references for cattle husbandry and their nutritional aspects. Persons had an undoubted extensive acceptance in Indian way of life and had chapters on diseases of human beings, horses, elephants, cattle and their treatments. The horse ayurved has two narrations, one by Dhanvantri and the other by Salihotra. HASTYA-AYRUVEDA, a work on husbandry and diseases of elephants, and "ASHVA-PARIKSHA", a work on husbandry and diseases of horses both in Sanskrit exist, though it is not known as to when these were first written.

Pre-Independence

The modern veterinary practice in India is traceble to the period of Moghul and Maratha Empires. East India Company, after virtually eclipsing the Moghul Empire in North and Maratha Empire in the Deccan in the later half of the eighteenth century, settled down to govern and administer the country in order to meet their remount needs. Some horse breeding farms were started in 1774 under the army establishment. In 1778, Joseph Earles got Sanskrit work on horse management and diseases translated into English and worked in consonance with it. Similar treatise was published by Pigott in Calcutta shortly afterwards. The army authorities were extremely anxious over the knotty problem of equine malady in 1793. Surprisingly there was not a single trained individual available in India who could be the doctor of horses.

Systematic livestock breeding and problems of animal health do not appear to have much concern for the European community in India much before the end of the eighteenth century. A non-veterinarian who had a profound influence on the development of livestock work, particularly horse-breeding in India, was Lieutenant William Frazer who proposed a plan for improvement of horses in 1793. In 1796, Coleman, Principal of the London Veterinary College, had undertaken to train medical men and others to serve as veterinary surgeons in the Army. The first commission to Veterinary Surgeons in H. M. Army was granted in 1797 and in 1799, five commissioned in H. M. Army arrived to join their regiments in India. They were Joseph Erratt, Thomas Burrows, James Grellier, Richard Davies and Samul Newman. By 1820, veterinary practitioners started arriving India in small numbers, and there was a general awakening of interest in the profession. The East India Company did not make similar appointments in their own Army until 1826. William Moorcroft was the first Veterinary Surgeon to be engaged in civilian capacity by the Company in 1808. Born at Ormskirk, Lancashire, in 1767, Moorcroft after his medical career at the Liverpool (UK), received training at the Veterinary School at Lyons. Moorcroft was not only a great explorer, ethnologist and ecologist, but was also a great veterinary surgeon. He left a profound impression on the veterinary field and refused headship at the London Veterinary School as he could not leave his profitable veterinary practice. His exploits gained early recognition for the profession in India, and he was one of the three outstanding men serving there in the nineteenth century; the others being J. H. B. Hallen and J. H. Steel, who contributed tremendously towards research, education and for the development of a Civil Veterinary Department. In India, too, the veterinary services were at a great disadvantage in being without their own administrative head. One was appointed in 1882; but in 1912 the Civil Veterinary Department came under the Agricultural Adviser and for yet another seventeen years there was no veterinarian at the Head of affairs. In 16 years, after his early resignation from the joint professorship with Coleman, he made a fortune for himself and later accepted an invitation from the East India Company in 1808, to become the Superintendent of their stud in Bengal on a salary of 3000/- per year. He diagnosed BURSATI and recorded its prevalence in Pusa (Bihar). He also drew attention to glanders, strangles, paraplegia and anthrax. He also described parasitic aneurysm of the mesenteric artery. Data on crop was introduced for feeding horse. He introduced a system of cooperative breeding with native stud farms.

The East India Company instructed J. T. Hodgson in 1821, who was attached as veterinary surgeon to the Governor-General's bodyguard in Calcutta, to arrange a course of instructions for eight apothecaries, who would later be employed with corps of Indian cavalry as sub-assistant Veterinary Surgeons. Hodgson objected to the plan and suggested only veterinary surgeons should be employed in the Company's service. The Government of India did not agree to his proposal, however, his proposal seemed to have given an impression in 1826 which expressed that the services of regular, educated Veterinary Surgeons in mounted corps will improve efficiency. As such, Hodgson himself was appointed first time to the Company's military service in 1826. In 1832 the Company insisted on a veterinary surgeon being appointed to the staff at various depots. J. T. Hodgson was evidently an able man and he pleaded for the organisation of a veterinary service for India. His scheme was sent to Coleman- at that time Princial Veterinary Surgeons to the British Army. Coleman pretended that creation of a post similar to his post may be a challenge for his own position, hence the scheme could not be materialised and the Compnay's Veterinary Department in India remained without any administrative officer for forty years.

East India Company Service-Recruitment

It is also interesting to note the procedure of recruitment of officers to the Company's service. An applicant having passed through the London College, was examined by the Board of Directors by a senior veterinarian in London, and for many years this duty was performed by William Sewell. Initially students passed out from London were taken but later students who passed out from Edinburgh were also accepted. After arriving in India, the newly appointed officer was again examined by a Board, consisting of two medical men and one veterinarian, before final acceptance by the Company. There were thirty-one officers for the three Presidencies of Madras, Bombay and Bengal in 1832. In 1853 the profession evidently grew restless over the want of a head of the Company's service in India. In 1859, a Royal Warrant was issued to improve the conditions of service of officers serving in the Army but for no obvious reasons, Government of India did not put the provisions of warrant into effect. Eventually, the

Bombay Government took upon itself to make a staff appointment, and J. H. B. Hallen, who had been made Superintendent of their Stud department in 1863, was appointed Principal Veterinary Surgeon in that presidency. This was followed in Bengal in 1866 and appointed two Inspecting Veterinary Surgeons. As a result of this pressure on the Government of India, R. J. G Hurford was appointed the first P.V. S. in India and the government simultaneously created posts of Inspecting Veterinary Surgeons in three presidencies.

Lord Harington, Secretary of State for India promulgated that the Department of Agriculture should pay careful attention to cattle diseases and comprehensive measures should be taken in cooperation with provincial government to deal with it. This set in motion an idea for the formation of Civil Veterinary Department. A committee was organised at Calcutta in 1883 which recommended the formation of a Civil Veterinary Department for the entire country. In May 1892 the Civil Veterinary Department finally came into existence.

Indian Plague Commission

Dr. K. McLeod, Civil Surgeon of Jessore published a report of his investigations on cattle in 1817 which referred severe epidemics in 1817 and fatal outbreak of rinderpest. McLeod referred to three important diseases in Bengal viz: foot and mouth disease (FMD), rinderpest (RP) and haemorrhagic septicaemia (HS). These reports put Government of India into action, for in 1869 they announced the appointment of an **Indian Cattle Plague Commission** with joint veterinary, medical and lay personnel. Col. J.H.B. Hallen first of its member, was appointed as the President of Indian Cattle Plague Commission and his colleagues were McLeod, A. C. Mangles, a Bengal civilian and babu Hem Chander Kerr. Originally, the Commission intended that enquiry should be restricted to Bengal, N. W. and Oudh, but the Commission later covered the whole of India. Both in a qualitative as well as a quantitative sense, the enquiry was an exhaustive one, and in addition to epidemic diseases dealt, supply of meat and milk to Calcutta, the hides industry, cattle poisoning, veterinary education and cattle breeding were also given attention. His pioneering work stimulated interest in veterinary work and several investigators took interest in diagnosis of obscure diseases like Bursati, *Lichen tropicus,* calcarious nodules in horses, anthrax, worm infection and paraplegia. Kumri received considerable attention from several workers including Queripal and Fedrick Smith.

The Commission's report of 1871 referred to special attention on the diseases as follows: rinderpest, foot and mouth disease, hoven, quarter ill, pleuro-pneumonia, purging, cystic disease and malignant sore throat (haemorrhagic septicaemia). A notable omission was that of Anthrax which was later given attention. The commission made the following recommendations:

1. When disease breaks out, it should be the subject of a special enquiry by committees or skilled agents.
2. An accurate census should be taken before and after the outbreak.
3. Systematic storage of fodder and preservation of pasture lands were important.
4. Herding and moving cattle during an outbreak should be regulated.
5. Large fairs should be subject to skilled inspection and sanitary precautions.
6. The hide trade is a source of danger and should be regulated.
7. Slaughter houses should be kept under skilled supervision.
8. A law should be enacted for the repression and prevention of the spread of disease.
9. A Government cattle should be placed under veterinary charge.
10. A veterinary school for the training of a skilled subordinate agency should be organised.
11. Such agents should be attached to municipalities and collaborate to investigate disease and apply preventive and remedial measures.
12. A yearly summary of all the information collected should be prepared and the preparation of this report should be the duty of some particular individual office or department.

A proposal to introduce legislation to prevent the spread of glanders and other contagious diseases was met with the reply that suitable action could be taken under the `nuisance' sections of the Indian Penal Code.

A great event in the history of Veterinary Science occurred when veterinary surgeon Griffith Evans announced discovery of *Trypanosoma evansi* as a causative agent of Surra in camels. Evans reported his discovery to the Adjutant General, Punjab Frontier Force, on 13 November 1880.

Hallen acted as a Veterinary Advisor for many years to Government of India before he was appointed Inspector-General, C. V. D. in 1982. The most outstanding contributions made during the time of Hallen were the establishment of the Imperial Bacteriological Laboratory at Muktehswar (Kumaon, UP), and a number of Veterinary Schools.

Imperial Bacteriological Laboratory

Indian Plague Commission led to the foundation stone of the Imperial Bacteriological Laboratory by the then Governor of Bombay, on 9th December 1889 at Poona (Pune) which was opened for the investigation of Surra in horses and camels. The name of this laboratory was changed as the Imperial Institute of Veterinary Research in 1925 and after the independence the name was rechrishtened as Indian Veterinary Research Institute (IVRI). Establishment of IVRI in pre-independence India show far sighteness of Britishers and it was a landmark in the history of veterinary science in the world. The details pertaining to IVRI will be described separately. In India, Dr. J. T. Edwards revolutionised preventive work against rinderpest. Rinderpest had been officially declared the most important disease entity of cattle in India and its control measures were taken up at the Imperial bacteriological Laboratory. It was felt that the climate in Poona was not suitable for intensive bacteriological studies, and for investigation of rinderpest a cooler and more secluded site was needed. Eventually, Mukteshwar in the Kumaon Hills used as an apple growing station by the United provinces was purchased. The laboratory moved from Poona to Mukteshwar in 1893. Further details about Mukteswar and Imperial Bacteriological laboratory are given under the description of Indian Veterinary Research Institute under the head Research Institutes in following pages.

Indian Civil Veterinary Department

In 1902, the Indian Civil Veterinary Department, later to be known as the Indian Veterinary Service, was firmly established with the permanent transfer of 17 officers from the Army Veterinary Department to the Civil Department.Four civil officers were recruited in India by the Secretary of State for India and this procedure of recruitment or local appointment remained in force till the end of British rule in India.

Post-Independence

After independence, further impetus in the progress of veterinary science and education took place throughout the length and breadth of India. Further expansion included establishment of veterinary colleges. Indian Veterinary Research Institute (IVRI) also took a lead by starting training programmes and diploma courses. Veterinary research became an affair of not only IVRI but also a part of teaching institutions under aegies of State Agricultural Universities.

The establishment of Veterinary Council of India (VCI) in 1984 is a great milestone. Now Veterinary Universities are coming up which should foster veterinary science in much better way. The ICAR having realised the future needs of veterinary science has been active in creation of institutes based on animal species. These institutes, besides other mandatory functions, will strengthen important animal species, in particular their conservation and development.

In the area of animal health and production numerous modern molecular techniques are now employed in the country. These include Embryo Transfer Technology (ETT), Recombinant-Genetic Engineering, Restriction Fragment Length Polymorphism (RFLP), Polymerase Chain Reaction (PCR). In a globally competitive scenario, efforts need to be continued to do little more than what has been achieved so far. The various details and milestones during post-independence have been described in independent sections wherever necessary.

Chapter - 4

INTERNATIONAL ORGANISATIONS

OFFICE INTERNATIONAL DES EPIZOOTIES

O. I. E. 12, Rue De Prony-75017, Paris, France

The office International des Epizooties was founded in 1924 to improve world-wide cooperation in controlling contagious animal diseases. There are now 111 member countries. The activities of the OIE are guided by an International Committee which meets at a General Session annually. The delegates are generally the Chief Veterinary Officers from each country. The OIE's most important role is to dessiminate information on epizootics which endanger livestock or pose a hazard to human health. OIE publishes several journals, monographs and conference proceedings.

COMMONWEALTH VETERINARY ASSOCIATION

Office: Commonwealth Veterinary Association "Galwiji" RMB N141, Scotsburn, Victoria, Australia 3352

Tel. (61 53) 41 3397

Fax (61 53) 41 2273

President: Dr. W.J. Pryor

Commonwealth Veterinary Association (CVA) was founded in 1970. Membership is open to national veterinary associations of Commonwealth member countries. Currently the CVA has 48 members with each member association being represented on a Regional Council by an elected Councillor. The aims and objectives as set out in CVA constitution are :

— To promote within the Commonwealth the interests of the veterinary and allied science.
— To maintain the honour and traditions of the profession.
— To effect the close possible links between member associations.
— To facilitate dissemination of professional knowledge and information.
— To encourage the creation of a national veterinary association in any Commonwealth member country where none exists.
— To promote interchange between its members.
— To encourage the creation of statutory bodies to regulate the study and practice of veterinary science in member countries where none exist.
— To promote animal health and welfare, and veterinary public health within the Commonwealth.
— Such other purpose as from time to time may be considered desirable by the Association.

CVA Councillor for India

Dr. S. Abdul Rahman

CVA Councillor, India &

Editor, CVA News

No.123, 7th B Main Road

IV Block (West) Jayanagar

BANGALORE- 560 011, India.

WORLD VETERINARY ASSOCIATION

Office: Dr. Lars Holsaae, Executive Secretary, World Veterinary Association, Rosenlunds Alle 8, 2720 Vanlose, Denmark

Ph + 45 38 7101 56

Fax +45 38 71 03 22

President: Dr. J.T. Blackburn (United Kingdom)

The World Veterinary Association (WVA) was founded in 1959 as a continuation of the Permanent Committee for the International Veterinary Congress, the first of which was held in Hamburg, Germany in 1863. WVA is a non political, non religious and non profit making association. Its objectives include:

— To unify the veterinary profession throughout the world
— To promote veterinary science and practice
— To encourage the setting of the highest possible standards
— To promote standards of health and welfare in all species of animal
— To organise World Veterinary Congress
— To defend the rights inherent of the veterinary diploma and to promote the standing of the profession
— To encourage the exchange of information of veterinary interest between the members
— To establish and maintain relations with other organisations whose interests are related to the objectives of the Association

INTERNATIONAL COUNCIL FOR LABORATORY ANIMAL SCIENCE

Secretary-General: University of Hanninen, University of Knopio, P.O. Box 6, SF-70211,

Knopio, Finland; Tel: +358-71-163080

On the initiative of the United Nations, UNESCO, the Council for International Organisations of Medical Science (CIOMS) and the International Union of Biological Sciences (IUBS), the International Committee on Laboratory Animals (ICLA) was conceived in 1956, as a non- governmental organisation to promote globally, high standards of laboratory animal, quality, care and health. In 1979 ICLA was renamed as International Council for Laboratory Animal Science (ICLAS). The Aims of the International Council for Laboratory Animal Science (ICLAS) are :

— To promote and coordinate the development of Laboratory Animal Science throughout the world.
— To promote international collaboration.
— To promote quality monitoring and definition of Laboratory Animals.
— To collect and disseminate information on Laboratory Animal Science.

— To promote the humane use of animals in research through recognition of ethical principles and scientific responsibilities.

In pursuing these objectives, ICLAS shall observe the basic policy of non-descrimination and affirm the rights of scientists throughout the world to adhere to, or to associate with, international scientific activity without regard to race, religion, political philosophy, ethnic origin, citizenship, language or sex. Following categories are available for ICLAS membership:

— National members, one per country, appointed by appropriate bodies concerned with the direction and encouragement of scientific research

— Scientific members, one representative appointed by Laboratory Animal Science Associations

— Associate members, one representative per organisation in sympathy with the aim of ICLAS and

— Union members, one representative per international non-governmental organisations such as International Scientific Unions.

WOLRD POULTRY SCIENCE ASSOCIATION (INDIA BRANCH)

Secretary, Dr. Ir, P. C. M. Simons, Centre for Applied Poultry Research, "Het Spelderholt" PB 31, 7360 AA BEEKBERGEN, THE NETHERLANDS, TEL:+31-55-5066534

President (India Branch): Dr. Anuradha Desai

Office: "Janaki", 189, Bhandarkar Road

Near Kamila Nehru Park, Pune-411 004 (Maharashtra)

Tel: 0212-371548, 376380

Fax No. 0212-371729

The World Poultry Science Association (WPSA) was founded on and its branch was opened in India in 1983. The objectives of the WPSA is to promote the advancement of knowledge of all aspects of Poultry Science and Poultry industry, to encourage regional poultry conferences, to cooperate with national and international organisations, to support the World's Poultry Science Journal and to create a library.

Chapter - 5

NATIONAL BODIES

DEPARTMENT OF ANIMAL HUSBANDRY & DAIRYING

Minsitry of Agriculture, Krishi Bhawan, Dr. Rajendra Prasad Road, New Delhi-11001Tel:(011) 3388911, 3382011; Gram : Agrindia; Telex:31-65054 AGRI IN; Fax:011-3388006.

The Department of Animal Husbandry, Ministry of Agriculture, Government of India is headed by Minister of State for Animal. Husbandry and Dairying (Independent Charge).

This department can be said a seat of Animal Husbandry Programmes throughout the country, including import and export of germ plasm, various biologicals and clearance for import of various vaccines, bacteria or other microorganisms, policy for slaughter houses. This department got a key post of Animal Husbandry Commissioner besides Secretary and other staff at different levels. This department envisages the following Divisions:

1. The Dairy Development Division
2. The Animal Husbandry Division

The Animal Husbandry Division is comprised of the following units/sections:

(i) Animal Husbandry Statistics

(ii) Livestock Feeds and Fodder

(iii) Livestock Health

(iv) National Project on Rinderpest Eradication (NPRE)

(v) Livestock Production

(vi) Livestock Extension

(vii) Meat and Meat products

(viii) Animal Quarantine and Certification Service Stations

(ix) National Informatics Centre

There are a number of other activities under the control of this division which includes:

Central Cattle Breeding Farms

Central Frozen Semen Production and Training Institute, Bangalore

Central Herd Registration Scheme, Ahemdabad

Central Fodder Seed production

The details of various farms and stations under the control of Department of Animal Husbandry and Dairying have been mentioned in subsequent pages.

VETERINARY COUNCIL OF INDIA (VCI)

Office: Veterinary Council of India, 16/15 W.E.A. Arya Samaj Road, Karol Bagh, New Delhi-110005, India.

Ph:011-5743804, 5750311, 5750323

Fax: 091-011-5743804

President: Dr. C.M. Singh

Secretary: Dr. Rama Kumar V

Veterinary Council of India (VCI) is a statutory body of the government of India established under the Indian Veterinary Council (IVC) Act , 1984 which was passed by both houses of Parliament and after receiving the assent of the President of India on 18th August, 1984. The Act envisaged estabiishment of VCI at the Centre and State Veterinary Councils in such states which had adopted the Indian Veterinary Council Act and in all Union territories of India. The VCI drew its insignia from the Ashoka era which projects the veterinary profession of India in its "best heritage". The sculpture of a bull and a part of the text of the stone edict are from the period of Emperor Ashoka (Around 300 B.C.). VCI chose a `Pali'script from IX rock edict which read on the fourth line `Panesu Saymo' [Barua B.M. (1955) Ashoka and his inscriptions, Calcutta]. The nearest meaning of which could be "compassion for animals".

Salient features and objectives of VCI are as follows:

(i) Lay down minimum standards of veterinary education required for granting recognised veterinary qualifications by veterinary institutions in those States to which this Act extends.

(ii) Recommend recognition or withdrawl of recognition of veterinary qualifications granted by veterinary institutions in India.

(iii) Maintain the Indian Veterinary Practitioners register which shall contain the names of all persons who possess the recognised veterinary qualifications and who are for the time being enrolled on a State Veterinary Register of the State to which IVC Act extends.

(iv) Lay down the standards of professional conduct, etiquette and code of ethics to be observed by veterinary practitioners.

(v) Negotiate with institutions located in other countries imparting training in veterinary education for recognition of their qualifications on reciprocal basis.

(vi) Advise both the Central and the State Governments, on all matters concerning veterinary education and practice

(vii) Only persons registered on the Indian Veterinary Practitioner's register would be entitled to practice veterinary medicine and to recover fees and charges in respect of medicaments and other appliances.

(viii) Only registered veterinary practitioners whose names are borne on Indian Veterinary Practioners register shall have the right to hold office as veterinary physician, surgeon or such similar position (by whatever name called), authenticate health certificates and give evidence under Indian Evidence Act, 1872, on matters relating to veterinary medicine. Veterinary practice by unregistered persons, would be prohibited except minor veterinary services, under supervision of a registered Veterinary practitioner, by 'specified' persons and as per the discretion of State Government (Section 30, IVC Act).

INDIAN COUNCIL OF AGRICULTURAL RESEARCH

Office: Krishi Bhavan, Dr. Rajendra Prasad Road, New Delhi-110001

Tel:011-3382629, Fax:91-11-3387293, E. mail: @ icar.delhi.nic.in

President: Honb'le Sh. Atal Behari Bajpai

Director-General : Dr. R.S. Paroda

National Bureaux : 4

Number of National Institutes: 4

Number of Research Institutes: 41

Number of National Research Centres: 30

Number of Project Directorates: 10

Number of All-India Coordinated Research projects: 86

Number of State Agricultural Universities (SAUs) supported: 29

Number of Central University : 1

Number of Deemed Universities: 4

In 1928, a Royal Commission was appointed to enquire into the conditions of agriculture and rural economy. The Commission proposed for the establishment of a Central Council of Agricultural Research to promote, guide and coordinate agricultural research throughout the country. In accordance with this recommendation, the Imperial Council of Agricultural Research was set up in 1929. The name of the Council was changed as the Indian Council of Agricultural Research (ICAR) in 1947.

ICAR is an autonomous body registered Society under the Registration of Societies Act XXI, 1860 and the officers of the society are : The Governing body, the Standing Finance Committee, Norms and Accredition Commitee, eight Regional Committee, Scientific Panels of the ICAR, the Joint Panels formed between the ICAR and related research organisations like CSIR, ICMR and ICSSR, the President of the Society, the Director-General of the Council, the Secretary of the Council and such other authorities/officers who may be appointed by the Governing Body or the Government of India.

The ICAR is an apex body responsible for the organisation and management of research and education in the fields of

Agriculture, Animal Sciences and Fisheries in India. The mandate of the Council are:

1. To plan, undertake, aid, promote and coordinate education, research and its application in agriculture, agroforestry, animal husbandry, fisheries, home science and allied sciences
2. To act as a clearing-house of research and general information relating to agriculture, animal husbandry, home science and allied sciences, and fisheries through its publications and information system, and instituting and promoting transfer of technology programmes.
3. To provide, undertake and promote consultancy services in the fields of education, research, training and dissemination of information in agriculture, agroforestry, animal husbandry, fisheries, home science and allied sciences.
4. To look into the problems relating to broader areas of rural development concerning agriculture, including post-harvest technology, by developing cooperative programmes with other organisations such as the Indian Council of Social Science Research, Council of Scientific and Industrial Research, Bhabha Atomic Research Centre, Universities.
5. To do other things considered necessary to attain the objectives of the Society

AGRICULTURAL SCIENTIST RECRUITMENT BOARD

(ASRB) Krishi Anusandhan Bhavan, Pusa, New Delhi-110012

Tel:011-5742295, 5766540; Gram:AGRECBOARD; Telex:031-77123 KAB IN; Fax:091-11-5766311

On the recommendations of Mr. Gajendragadkar committee in 1972 and on examination by a group of Ministers headed by Minister of Agriculture by Government in 1973, it was recommended to initiate a recruitment procedure through a special Agricultural Scientist Recruitment Board with an eminent agricultural scientists as a whole-time Chairman. Initial induction through an all-India competitive examination and interviews were conducted by ASRB in March 1976 for Scientists to be recruited under Agricultural Research Service (ARS). Since then ASRB has been conducting examinations for scientists and administrative posts through competitions. Now the ASRB is also conducting an all-India examination for National Eligibility Test (NET). In addition, ASRB is recruiting scientists at higher levels by direct advertisements.

UTTAR PRADESH COUNCIL OF AGRICULTURAL RESEARCH

Office: 16, A.P. Sen Road, Charbagh, Lucknow-226001 (UP)

Tel: (O) 0522-451136, 458325, 452367, 454146; Fax:0522-456315

Director General : Dr. S.C. Moudgal

Uttar Pradesh Council of Agricultural Research (UPCAR) was established in July 1989 as a registered society under Society Registration Act 21, 1860 to coordinate research, education and extension activities in the State Agricultural Universities, Government Departments and other organisations of agricultural institutions engaged in the fields of agriculture, horticulture, animal sciences, fisheries, natural resources management and allied disciplines.

CENTRAL ZOO AUTHORITY

Barrack No.4, Bikaner House, Shahajahan Road

New Delhi-110011

The Government of India amended Wild Life (Protection) Act in September 1991 and brought the management of the zoos under the purview of this act. The Central Zoo Authority was constituted on 3rd february 1992 to oversee and monitor the management of zoos in the country in such a manner that they contribute significantly in the *ex-situ* conservation of rare and endangered species. The responsibilities assigned to the Central. Zoo Authority under the Wild Life (protection) Act include specification of minimum standards for housing, upkeep and veterinary care of the animals kept in a zoo, evaluation and functioning of zoos with respect to the standards, identification of endangered species of wild animals for purposes of captive breeding and assigning responsibility, coordination for the exchange of zoo animals, training of zoo personels and other such assistance to zoos.

ANIMAL WELFARE BOARD OF INDIA

2nd Cross Street, Venus Colony,Alwarpet, Madras-600 018 (TN)
Tel:455819

The Animal Welfare Board of India is aimed for the animal welfare, education, animal welfare training, prevention of exploitation of animals and cruelty free society. The Board organises seminars and courses to dessiminate its objectives. It also publishes a popular magazine "*Animal Citizen.*

Chapter - 6

ACADEMIES

THE NATIONAL ACADEMY OF SCIENCES IN INDIA

5, Lajpat Rai Road, Allahabad-211002 (UP)

Tel:0531-640224; Fax:0532-641183; Gram:NATACADEMY

Founded in the year 1930, the National Academy of Sciences India is the oldest Science Academy of the country. The main objective of the Academy is to provide a national forum for the publication of research work carried out by Indian scientists and to provide opportunities for exchange of views among them. The Rules and Regulations of the Academy are based on those of the Royal Society of England and Asiatic Society of Bengal. Since its inception, the Academy publish two quarterly journals-Proceedings of the National Academy of Sciences (Section A-Physical Science) and the Proceedings of the National Academy of Sciences, India (Section B-Biological Sciences). Since 1978, it is also publishing a monthly journal, the National Academy Science Letters (monthly) for speedy publication of important research work. The Academy also holds seminars, symposia etc.

INDIAN NATIONAL SCIENCE ACADEMY (INSA)

1, Bahadur Shah Zafar Marg, New Delhi-110 002

Fax:91-11-3235648 and 91-11-3231095

E. mail:insa@giasdlo1.vsn.net.in and insa@delnet.ren.nic.in

The Indian National Science Academy was established in January 1935 with an object to promote science in India and to harness scientific knowledge for the cause of humanity and national welfare. The Academy promotes scientific knowledge, coordination between scientific bodies and safeguards the interests of scientists in India and adhering to organisation of ICSU. The Academy publishes Proceedings, Monographs, Bulletins, Progress of Science in India, Indian Journal of History of Science, Year book, Indian Journal of Pure and Applied Mathematics, Biographical Memoirs and recently in 1997 introduced a review journal.

INDIAN ACADEMY OF SCIENCES

CV Raman Avenue, POB 8005, Sadashivanagar, Bangalore-560080

Tel:080-3344592; Telex:845-2178; Fax:080-3346094.

The Academy publishes Proceedings Chemical Sciences (every 2 months), Proceedings Earth and Planetary Sciences (quarterly), Pramana (journal of Physics, monthly), Journal of Bioscience, Journal of Astrophysics and Astronomy (quarterly), Bulletin of Materials Science (every 2 months), Sadhana (Engineeering Sciences, every two months), Journal of Genetics (quarterly), resonance (monthly), Current Science (fortnightly), Patrika (news letter), Year Book.

NATIONAL ACADEMY OF AGRICULTURAL SCIENCES (NAAS)

Avenue II, Indian Agricultural Research Institute
Campus, New Delhi-110012
Tel:011-5753677, 5753713
Fax:091-11-5753678.

The National Academy of Agricultural Sciences (NAAS) concerned with crop husbandry, animal husbandry, fisheries, forestry, agroindustries and allied sciences was founded in 1990 under the Society Registration Act, 21 of 1860 with the following major objectives:

* to promote ecologically sustainable agriculture
* to recognise and support excellence in scientific research in the field of agriculture performed by the individual scientists and by interdisciplinary teams
* to provide promising scientists with conditions necessary for the advancement of their work

* to promote contact among research workers in different institutions and organisations within the country and with the world scientific community
* to secure and manage funds and endowments for the promotion of agricultural sciences
* to publish documents and specific studies including those intended for policy makers for the advancement of agricultural research and development
* other activities relevant to the accomplishment of the above goals in public interest

The membership of the Academy is constituted by Fellows elected by the Academy. In addition scientists with outstanding contributions in the field of Agricultural Research are invited to become Fellows of the Academy.

NATIONAL ACADEMY OF VETERINARY SCIENCES

16/15 W. E. A. Arya Samaj Road, Karol Bagh, New Delhi-110 006Tel:011-5743804, 5750311, 5750323; Fax:011-5743804

President: Dr. C. M. Singh

On the lines of Medical Council of India, National Academy of Veterinary Sciences was created in 1996. The Academy was inaugurated by Honb'le Dr. Raghuvansh Prasad Singh, Minister of Animal Husbnadry & Dairying (Independent charge) on 18-12-1996. One hundred veterinarians were nominated as its Fellows authorizing them to use the title "FNAVSc". 80% of the nominated Fellows were above 60 years of age and 10 Fellows from abroad were also included. The modalities of this FNAVSc are under process of preparation.

NATIONAL ACADEMY OF AGRICULTURAL RESEARCH MANAGEMENT (NAARM)

Rajendra Nagar, Hyderbad-500 030 (AP)Tel:040-4015070; Telex: 04256651 STAG IN; Fax:245912; Gram:STAFFAGRI, E-mail @ x 400 nicgw. nic. in. naarm.

Director: Dr. J. C Katyal

The National Commission on Agriculture (NCA) recommended the establishment of an all India institute for administration and management in agriculture. The National Academy of Agricultural Research Management (NAARM), earlier known as Central Staff College of Agriculture, was thus set up in 1976 as one of the constituent institutions of the Indian Council of Agricultural Research (ICAR) under the aegis of the Department of Agriculture Research and Education (DARE), Ministry of Agriculture, Govt. of India. The Academy since its inception, has been assisting the deemed- to- be universities, research institutes of the ICAR and the State Agricultural Universities (SAUs) by providing training input for management of agricultural research, education, training and extension.

Chapter - 7

RESEARCH INSTITUTES

Consolidated list of ICAR Research Institutes/Centres

Sl.No.	*Institute*	*Establishment Year*
1.	Indian Veterinary Research Institute	1889
2.	National Dairy Research Institute	1955
3.	Central Sheep & Wool Research Institute	1962
4.	Central Avian Research Institute	1979
5.	Central Institute for Research on Goats	1979
6.	National Research Centre on Camels	1984
7.	National Institute of Animal Genetics	1984
8.	National Bureau of Animal Genetic Resources	1984
9.	Central Institute for Research on Buffaloes	1985
10.	National Research Centre on Equines	1986
11.	National Research Centre on Mithun	1988
12.	National Research Centre on Yak	1989
13.	National Institute of Animal Nutrition and Physiology	1995

INDIAN VETERINARY RESEARCH INSTITUTE

Izatnagar-243 122, BAREILLY (UP) Tel:0581-447069,447684 ; Gram: VETEX; Fax:0581-447284 E.mail:IVRI@x400.nicgw nic in

Year of establishment :	1889
Livestock Health Divisions	12
Livestock Production Divisions	4
Basic and Social Science Divisions	4

Livestock Products Technology Division 1
Sections 10
Centres 5
Regional Stations & Campuses
Livestock Production Research (LPR) 1
on Cattle & Buffalo 1
LPR on pigs
LPR-Cattle, Goat, Laboratory Animals 1
All-India Coordinated Research Projects (AICRPs), AICRP on Epidemiological studies on Foot & Mouth Disease AICRP on Haemoprotista AICRP on Pigs.

The Indian Veterinary Research Institute (IVRI) owes a great historic importance in the country. It has played an yeoman service in the organisation of veterinary research and education in India.

Historical Perspective
Pre-independence

Preliminary work on the diagnosis of diseases in ancient and pre-independence India was undertaken. Britishers having realized the importance of rendering a proper laboratory investigations, the John Company brought British veterinarians in 1917 to undertake work on tropical diseases. These workers did not possess sufficient knowledge to undertake investigation of animal diseases. Thus, Indian Plague Commission was set up in 1869 to study the devastating plague in Indian and British colonies. The deliberations of this commission led to the foundation of the `Imperial Bacteriological Laboratory' on 5.5 acres of land donated by a Parsi Philanthropist, Sir Dinshaw Manockji Petit, at Poona. The foundation stone was laid down by the then Governor of Bombay on 9 December 1889. The mandate of the laboratory was:

"To investigate diseases of domesticated animals in all province of India and to ascertain as far as possible by biological research both in the laboratory and when necessary, at the place of outbreak, the means of preventing and curing such diseases."

This was the first scientific research laboratory of its own kind in India and probably in the East. Since modern refrigration techniques were unknown in those days, the climatic conditions of Pune were not conducive for research work. Location of the laboratory adjacent to populous part of the city was also a constraint for taking work on highly infectious diseases of cattle. Therefore, after a sojourn of two years, the laboratory was shifted in 1893 to a picturesque locale of Mukteswar (about 7,700 ft. above sea level with a temperature of 17-87^{0}F). The hilly topography, lush green surroundings and salubrious climate provided an excellent working condition.

On the recommendation of Dr.Theodar Cook, Principal College of Science, Poona, Dr. Alfred Lingard, was appointed in 1890 as Head of of the Imperial Bacteriological Laboratory. Two noted German Bacteriologists namely Robert Koch and Pfeiffer arrived at the laboratory to advise methods for cultivating and preparation of biologicals. It will not be an exaggeration in saying that Dr. Lingard was the real source of inspiration to research workers who having not bothered for his personal comforts and self interest served the laboratory in the Himalayan region amongst not only illiterate hilly people but also far from civil amenities. With the expansion of research activities at Mukteswar, it was found necessary to open a branch laboratory to study certain infections under "plain" conditions. A branch laboratory was opened in 1901 at Kargana, Bareilly (Uttar Pradesh) about 3 miles away from the Bareilly city. Later, in 1913, a suitable site was acquired at Izatnagar (Bareilly) for large scale manufacture of the sera and vaccines. In 1925, the Imperial Bacteriological Laboratory was given the title of "Imperial Institute of Veterinary Research." In 1936, the Imperial Veterinary Serum Institute, Izatnagar issued several biologicals against infectious diseases to fulfil the proverb "Prevention is better than cure" and subsequently, became the Biological Products Section of the Imperial Veterinary Research Institute. The Divisions of Animal Nutrition and Poultry Research were established by the then Viceroy and Governor-General of India, Lord Linlithgow in 1939. Some of the landmark research contributions made by the IVRI till 1947 are listed below:

* 1893- Relocated to Mukteswar-Kumaon (UP) from Pune
* 1897- Bile method of protection against Rinderpest

* 1897- Historic visit of Prof. Robert Koch, Prof. R. Pfeiffer and Prof. G. Gaffiky
* 1898- Dr. Leonard Rogers discovered role of tabanid flies in the transmission of Surra
* 1899- Anti-rinderpest serum
* 1902- Anti-anthrax serum for cattle
* 1904- First training programme to field veterinarians
* 1905- Haemorrhagic septicaemia serum
* 1906- Black Quarter vaccine
* 1907- Production of anti-rinderpest serum
* 1908- Treatment of Surra in horses
* 1913- Izatnagar campus came into existence
* 1927- Goat Tissue Rinderpest Vaccine developed
* 1936- Anthrax spore vaccine
* 1940- Ranikhet Disease virus vaccine
* 1942- First systematic work on Artificial Insemination
* 1947- Rechristened as Indian Veterinary Research Institute

After independence of India in 1947, the name of the institute was re-christened as the "Indian Veterinary Research Institute." A list of eminent workers who headed the IVRI during pre and post independence period is as follows:

Name(s)	Year(s)
Dr.Alfred Lingard	1890-1907
Sir Leonard Rogers*	1898-1900
Lt.Col. J.D.E Holmes	1907-1915
Dr. A.W. Shilston*	1915-1916
Dr.A.L. Sheather	1916-1920
Mr. W. A. Pool*	1920-1921
Dr. J. T. Edwards	1921-1929
Mr. H. Cooper*	1929
Mr.(Sir) Frank Ware	1929-1938
Mr. W. Taylor	1937-1938
Dr.J.R. Haddow*	1938-1939
Dr.F.C. Minett	1939-15th August 1947

Contd....

Dr. G. D. Bhalerao*	1947
Dr. S. Datta	1947-1954

Name(s)	Year(s)
Dr. Lakshmi Sahai	1954-1957
Dr. N.D. Kher*	1957-1958
Dr. P.G. Pandey	1958-1961
Dr.H.D. Srivastava*	1961-1963
Dr.M.R. Dhanda*	1963-1966
Dr.C.M. Singh	1966-1982
Dr. B.S. Rajya*	1982-1984
Dr.P.N. Bhat	1984-14.8.1991; 4.5.1992
Dr. B. B. Mallick*	10.3.1991
Dr. O. N. Kunzru*	11.3.1991-13.8.1991
Dr. D. S. Balain*	4.5.1992-22.11.1994
Dr. G. C. Mohanty	31.3.1995-30.11.1995
Dr. P. N. Khanna*	1.12.1995- 26.12.1995
Dr. Kiran Singh*	27.12.1995 to Aug 1997
Dr. O. S. Tomar*	Aug 1997
Dr. Nagendra Sharma	19 April 1999

* Officiating Director

Siginificant post-independence research contributions of the IVRI are summarised as follows:

* 1950- Contagious ecthyma was reported first time and contagious caprine pleuropneumonia vaccine developed.
* 1958- Establishment of Postgraduate College of Animal Science
* 1960-64 Control and eradication of African Horse Sickness
* 1965- Kid kidney inactivated Foot and Mouth vaccine
* 1966- Administrative Control Transferred to ICAR
* 1967-68 Developed Tissue Culture Rinderpest vaccine
* 1969- Lungworm irradiated vaccine
* 1971- All India Coordinated Research Project on Foot and Mouth Disease at Mukteswar
* 1972- All India Coordinated Research Project on Pashmina Goat

* 1974 Quail an alternate to poultry was introduced first time in India
* 1977- A high yielding broiler strain (B-73) developed
* 1978- Development of BHK 21 inactivated Foot & Mouth vaccine
* 1979- *Theileria* schizont vaccine developed
* 1979- Large scale manufacture of monovalent and polyvalent FMD vaccine
* 1979- Poultry Research Department upgraded as an independent Central Avian Research Institute, Izatnagar
* 1983- Deemed University Status Conferred to IVRI
* 1986- Establishment of National Biotechnology Centre
* 1986-87 Goat-pox and sheep pox vaccines developed.
* 1990- First Convocation of Deemed University* 1999- Fourth Convocation of Deemed University

In fact, Veterinary Research is taking a rapid stride in the present era from 1980 onwards, much of the current research in biotechnology, immunology and molecular biology has been planned to bring about applicable results. IVRI at its Bangalore centre has evolved a sub-unit vaccine against A_{22} and ASIA-1 strains. In order to strengthen work both in research, education and extension, IVRI has opened regional centres.

IVRI Campuses

MUKTESHWAR

Joint Director & Incharge : Dr. P.C. Harbola

Address : Indian Veterinary Research Institute, Izatnagar, Kumaon Distt. : Nanital (UP), India.

Year of Establishment : 1893 the "Imperial Bacteriological Laboratory"

The campus now house Division of Virology, Livestock Production Research Centre and Foot and Mouth Centre.

BANGALORE

Joint Director & Incharge: Dr. L.D. Mishra

Address: Indian Veterinary Research, Hebbal, Banaglore-(Karnataka).

Year of Establishment : 1971

The campus was created with Danish collaboration for the large scale production of tissue culture Foot and Mouth (FMD) vaccine using fermentor technology. The campus also undertakes diagnosis, monitoring and surveillance of various diseases in the Southern region.

PALAMPUR

Incharge: Dr. B. Singh

Address: Indian Veterinary Research Institute, Regional Station, Palampur- (Himachal Pradesh), India.

Year of Establishment : 1969

Lays major emphasis on nutritional research of locally available feed resources and disease investigation of various health problems prevalent in the region.

SRINAGAR

Year of Establishment : 1972

The regional station gives major emphasis on irridiated lungworm vaccine, besides rendering diagnostic and advisory services. The centre is presently housed at Mukteshwar campus.

CALCUTTA

Incharge: Dr. Asim Sikdar

Address: Indian Veterinary Research Institute, Regional Station, 37, Belgachia, Calcutta- (West Bengal)

Year of Establishment : 1970

The major mandate of this regional station is to conduct Master's degree programme in veterinary Public Health, and to deal research problems of animal health in rural areas.

BHUBNESWAR

Incharge: Late Dr. D. Ramarao

The station was established in 1991. The objectives were to identify animal health problems, their diagnosis using modern diagnostic techniques including forecasting of diseases with the idea to provide health coverage to the state of Orissa for the control and prevention of diseases. The station was however closed.

BHOPAL

HIGH SECURITY ANIMAL DISEASES LABORATORY (HSADL)
Hathai Kheda Farm, Kokla Road, Anand Nagar, Bhopal-462 021 (MP).
Tel:0755-589204; Fax:0755-588842; Gram: VETEX, BHOPAL
Joint Director & Incharge: Dr. H.K. Pradhan

This laboratory was created with the assistance of 5.29 Crore by the World Bank to handle exotic and emerging diseases like bovine viral diarrhoea and caprine arthritis. The assistance also envisaged provision for structural equipments, laboratory equipments, training and consultancy.

IVRI PORT BLAIR UNIT

The IVRI unit of Port Blair established in 1970, for carrying out studies on stephanofilarial dermatitis, has since been merged with Central Agricultural Research Institute, Port Blair due to administrative reasons.

NATIONAL DAIRY RESEARCH INSTITUTE

Karnal-132 001 (Haryana) Tel:21611; Telex:0396-204 NDRI IN; Grams:DAIRYSEARCH
Year of Establishment : 1955
Director : Dr. O. S. Tomer

The majo⁻ focus of the institute is to undertake and promote basic and applied research in the areas of dairy production, technology, economics and extension marketing. To act as a centre of excellence to impart education and training and as such the institute has got a "Deemed University Status". Major programmes of the institute include germplasm collection of milch animals, embryo transfer technology, studies on post-partum anestrus and dairy products.

CENTRAL SHEEP AND WOOL RESEARCH INSTITUTE

Address: Avikanagar (Malpura Distt: Tonk)(Via Jaipur) Rajasthan-304 501 Gram: Sheep INST MALPURA Te: 0143-28145, Fax: 0143-28163

Year of Establishment : 1962

Director : **Dr. R. N. Singh**

The institute is engaged in research on various disciplines relating to sheep and rabbit production and their product utilization. The thrust areas include improving carpet wool production, apparel wool production, mutton, utilization of crop residues, cryopreservation of rams semen and embryotransfer technology in sheep.

CENTRAL AVIAN RESEARCH INSTITUTE

Izatnagar-243 122 (UP), India

Ph:0581-447261,447293 (R); EPBAX: 447223, 446420,Fax:091-581-447321, Telex:0577-206 CARI IN; E.mail: cavri @x400.nic gw.nic.in

Year of Establishment : 1979

Director : **Dr. Rajvir Singh**

The major mandate of the institute is to undertake basic and applied research in all disciplines to avian production and post harvest technology, to conserve, maintain and improve avian germplasm,to develop, update and standardise package of practices concerning feeding, management and health cover of poultry, referral and consultancy services.

CENTRAL INSTITUTE FOR RESEARCH ON GOATS

Makhdoom, P. O. Farah -281 122 Mathura (UP), India.

Tel: 0565-404810, 793246; Fax:0565-79-3246; Gram:VETEXFARAH; E. mail cirg @ X 400. nicgw. nic. in

Year of Establishment : 1979

Director : **Dr. K.P. Pant**

The Institute's mandate is to undertake basic and applied research, updating and standardizing area-specific package of practices concerning feeding, management, breeding and health-cover of goats.

NATIONAL RESEARCH CENTRE ON CAMEL

Jorbeer P.O. Shiv Keri, Bikaner 334 001 (Rajasthan), IndiaTel:0151-522183, 528858, 529070, 523187 27628, 25683; Fax:151-522183; Gram: CAMELNTRE BIKANERE. E.mail nrccamel@ 400.nicgwnic.in

Year of Establishment : 1984

Director : Dr. M. S. Sahani

Basic and applied research, repository of information on camel research and development, to coordinate and collaborate camel research with national and international agencies and to offer consultancy.

NATIONAL INSTITUTE OF ANIMAL GENETICS

NDRI Campus, Karnal-132 001 (Haryana), India.

Year of Establishment : 1984

Director : Dr. Rajendra Sahai

The institute conducts basic and applied research in population genetics, cytogenetics, immunogenetics (blood group), biochemical and molecular genetics, gene-marker characters and undertakes training programmes.

NATIONAL BUREAU OF ANIMAL GENETIC RESOURCES

NDRI Campus, Karnal- 132 001 (Haryana).

Year of Establishment : 21 September 1984

Director : Dr. A.E. Nivasarkar

The institute undertakes work on identification, description, evaluation and conservation of indigenous animal genetic resources, conservation and management of animal genetic resources, to develop animal genetic resource data-bank and gene bank and to impart training.

CENTRAL INSTITUTE FOR RESEARCH ON BUFFALOES

Sirsa Road, Hisar- 125 001 (Haryana), India Ph: 01662-38821, 39604 (R) 36490, 33147, 63170, Grams: BUBALINEX; Fax:01662-39604 ; E. mail cirb@x400nicgw nic.in

Year of Establishment : 1985

Director : **Dr. R. K. Sethi**

The institute's major mandate is to undertake research, to establish nucleus breeding herds, to act as a repository of information on all aspects of buffalo production and development and to undertake technology transfer activities.

NATIONAL RESEARCH CENTRE ON EQUINES

Sirsa Road, Hisar-125 001 (Haryana), India.

Tel:(O)01662-32787, 32748 (R):32955; FAX:01662-33217; E.MAIL:nrcequine @x400. nicgw.nic.in; Gram:EQUINE

Year of Establishment : 1986

Director : **Dr. M. P. Yadav**

A referral centre on equine research undertakes basic and applied research on equine health and production, development of vaccines and diagnostic technologies, repository centre for information, acts as a collaborating centre for other agencies, offers consultancy and advisory services.

NATIONAL RESEARCH CENTRE ON MITHUN

Jhamapani-797 106 (Nagaland)

Year of Establishment : 1988

Director : **Dr. N. D. Verma**

The Centre aims to improve mithun for meat and milk through selection and cross breeding with exotic and native cattle and to investigate nutritional and management aspects of mithun production including diseases.

NATIONAL RESEARCH CENTRE ON YAK

Dirang, West Kameng 790 101 (Arunachal Pradesh)

Year of Establishment : 1989

Director : **Dr. B. P. S. Yadav**

The Centre aims collection of germplasm and data base compilation including research on yak production, training and extension.

NATIONAL INSTITUTE OF ANIMAL PHYSIOLOGY & NUTRITION

NDRI Campus, Adugogi, Bangalore-560 030 (Karnataka) Tel: 5711303; (Res):2242924, Fax:080-5711420'

Mail:director@ nainpbng.Kar.nic.in

Year of establishment : 24 November 1995

Director : **Dr. Khub Singh**

This is newly established institute whose main focus will be to undertake research and training in the area of animal physiology and nutrition. This will include unraveling basic physiology and nutritional principles and conducting research on demonstrating how nutrition and physiology principles function in practice and thereby improve rural economy through better livestock feeding and management approaches.

Chapter - 8

INSTITUTES OTHER THAN THE ICAR

WILDLIFE INSTITUTE OF INDIA

P.O. Box-18, Chandrabani, Dehradun (UP)-248001

Director : Dr. S. K. Mukherjee

The major objectives of the Institue include:

* Training managers and biologists for protected area management and wildlife research
* Training education and extension specialists for protected areas to get public support for wildlife conservation
* Providing orientation courses for those involved in land use management
* Conducting and coordinating applied wildlife research and evolving relevant techniques suited to Indian conditions
* Creating a database for building up a wildlife information system employing modern analytical techniques and computer equipment
* Providing advisory and consultancy services to central and state governments, universities, research institutions, other official and non-official agencies
* Courses offered: Post-Graduate Diploma in Wildlife Management *Certificate in Wildlife Management, short term courses, trainings, workshop.

DEPARTMENT OF ANIMAL HUSBANDRY & DAIRYING

(Source: Directory of R&D Institutions, 1994, Deptt. of Science & Technology, New Delhi)

1. Central Cattle Breeding Farm, Andeshnagar-262 701 Dist: Lakhimpur Kheri (UP)
2. Central Cattle Breeding Farm, Hessarghatta, Bangalore-560 088 (Karnataka)
3. Central cattle Breeding Farm, Godhbhaga (Via), Basantpur (PO), Chiplima-768 111, Dist: Sambalpur.
4. Central cattle Breeding Farm, Dharmroda-394 125, Dist: Surat (Gujarat).
5. Central Cattle Breeding Farm, Avadi (Alamadhi), Red hills, Madras-600 052, Tami Nadu
6. Central Cattle Breeding Farm, Sunabeda, Semiliguda-763 002, Dist: Koraput (Orissa)
7. Central Cattle Breeding Farm, Suratgarh-335 804 Dist: Ganganagar (Rajasthan)
8. Central Duck Breeding Farm, Hessarghatta, Bangalore-560 088
9. Central Fodder Seed Production Farm, Hessarghatta, Bangalore- 560 088
10. Central Frozen Semen Production & Training Institute, Hessarghatta, Bangalore-560 088
11. Central Herd Registration Scheme, 10, Gautam Vihar, Cooperative Housing Society, Usmanpura, Ahemdabad (Gujarat)
12. Central Herd Registration Scheme, Christian Ganj, Ramble Road, Ajmer, Rajasthan
13. Central Herd Registration Scheme, 52/1/2/12, Bakergarden, Kapadipalem, Ongole-523 001 (AP)
14. Central Poultry Breeding Farm, Hessarghatta, Bangalore-560 088
15. Central Poultry Breeding Farm, Bhubneswar-751012 (Orissa)
16. Central Poultry Breeding Farm, Aarey Milk Colony, Bombay-400 065.

17. Central Poultry Breeding Farm, Industrial Area, Chandigarh- 160 002
18. Central Poultry Training Institute, Hessarghatta, Bangalore-560 088
19. Central Sheep Breeding Farm, P. O. Box. 10, Hisar-125 001 (Haryana)
20. Regional Feed Analytical Laboratory, Bhubneswar-751 012 (Orissa)
21. Regional Feed Analytical Laboratory, Aarey Milk Colony, Bombay-400 065 (MS)
22. Regional feed Analytical Laboratory (CPBF Campus), Industrial Area, Chandigarh-160 002
23. Regional Station for Forage Production & Demonstration, P.O. Textile Mill, Hissar-125 002
24. Regional Station for Forage Production & Demonstration, GH- 128/2, sector No.30, Gandhinagar-382 030.
25. Regional Station for Forage production & Demonstration, Mamidipally, Keshavagiri, Hyderabad-500 005 (AP)
26. Regional Station for Forage Production & Demonstration Camp Office, 599-A, Gandhi Nagar, Jammu-180 004 (J&K)
27. Regional Station for Forage production & Demonstration, Netaji Subhash Sanitorium, Kalyani-741 251, Dist: Nadia (WB)
28. Regional Station for Forage Production & Demonstration, Avadi (Alamadhi), cattle Farm (PO), Madras- 600 052 (TN)
29. Regional Station for Forage production & demonstration, Suratgarh-335 804 Dist:Sri Ganganagar (Rajasthan)

STATE GOVERNMENT INSTITUTES

(Source: Directory of R&D Institutions, 1994, Deptt. of Science & Technology, New Delhi).

The various state institutes have now been placed under different state universities.

Andhra Pradesh

1. Institute of Animal reproduction, Maandapeta-553 308 Distt: East Godavari

2. Livestock Research Station, Kondapuram Mandalam Kaligiri (Via) Chintaladevi-524 224 Distt:Nellore
3. Livestock Research Station, Garividi-532 101Dist: Viziangaram
4. Livestock Research Station, Lam-522 034 Dist: Guntur
5. Livestock Research Station, Palamaner-517 408, Dist: Chitoor
6. Poultry Research Institute, Rajendranagar, Hyderabad-500 030
7. Veterinary Biological and Research Institute, Shantinagar Hyderabad-500 028.

Assam

1. Goat Research Station, Burnihat-793 101, Dist: Kamrup
2. Livestock Research Station, Mandira, Barpeta-781 301

Bihar

1. Animal Production Research Institute, Birauli, Digha (PO) Waini-848 131 Dist: Darbhanga

Gujarat

1. Livestock Research Station, GAU Campus, Anand-388 110
2. Livestock Research Station, Navsari Campus, Navsari-396 450
3. Poultry Complex, GAU Campus, Anand-388 110 Dist: Kheda

Himachal Pradesh

1. Angora Rabbit Breeding Farm, Palampur-176 061, Dist: Kangra
2. Jersey Cattle Breeding Farm, Palampur-176 061 Dist: Kangra
3. Sheep Breeding Farm, Jeori-172 101, Dist: Shimla

Jammu & Kashmir

1. Exotic Cattle Breeding Farm, Mansbal
2. Sheep Breeding Farm, Shuhama

Kerala

1. Cattle Breeding Farm, Thumburmuzhi, Chalakudy-680 721
2. Livestock Research Station, Thiruvazhakunnu
3. Pig Breeding Farm, Mannuthy-680 651

Maharashtra

1. Animal Nutrition Research Centre, Aarey Goregaon (E), Mumbai- 400 065.
2. Cattle Breeding Farm, Borgaon-Manju Dist: Akola
3. Cattle Breeding Farm, Igatpuri-422 403 Dist: Nasik
4. Cattle Breeding Farm, Nileli-416 520

Orissa

1. Animal Disease Research Institute, Phulnakhara-754 001, Dist:Cuttack

Rajasthan

1. Livestock Research Station, Chandan-345 029, Dist: Jaisalmer
2. Livestock Research Stations, Vallabhnagar-313 601, Dist: Udaipur

Tamil Nadu

1. Centre for Animal Health Studies, Madhavaram Milk Colony, Madras-600 051
2. Livestock R&D Centre, 47, Samiappa Street, Thiru Nagar Colony, Erode-638 003
3. Poultry R &D Centre, Veterinary Hospital, Kamaraj Road, Tirupur-638 604
4. Poultry R & D Centre, Navaloor Kuttapattu, Tiruchirappalli-620 009
5. Poultry R & D Centre, Vamban-622 303
6. Poultry R & D Centre, 11, New Sankarapalayam Road, Vellore- 632 001 Dist: North Arcot
7. Poultry Research Station, Nandanam, Madras-600 035
8. Sheep Breeding Research Station, Sandynallah-643 237 Dist: Nilgiri
9. Sheep & Research Development Centre, Kovilangulam-626107

Chapter - 9

VETERINARY UNIVERSITIES

INDIAN VETERINARY RESEARCH INSTITUTE

DEEMED UNIVERSITY, IZATNAGAR-243 122 (UP)

Tel:0581-447069; Fax No: 0581-447284

Year of Establishment : November 1983

Chancellor : Union Minister of Agriculture

Vice-Chancellor : Director, IVRI

The Indian Veterinary Research Institute (IVRI) established in 1889, is India's premier institute solely devoted to research, education and extension in Veterinary and Animal Sciences. The institute first organised a training programme for field veterinarians from civil/army/other departments was started in 1904. Later, these programmes were rearranged in the form of National Diplomas. In 1943, the institute started the Associateship programme which was then recognised as equivalent to Master's degree. The postgraduate education and training were further strengthened by the establishment of P.G. college in 1958. In recognition of the Institute's past glorious contributions for the man power development, the institute was conferred the status of Deemed University in 1983. The first trimester of the last academic session started on 15.1.1985. The University has now adopted the semester system of education from 1994. The university offers Master's programme in 22 disciplines, Doctoral programme in 21 disciplines and National Diploma of 10 months duration in 9 disciplines.

TAMIL NADU VETERINARY AND ANIMAL SCIENCES UNIVERSITY

Madhavaram, Chennai-600 051

Phone (O)0091-44-5371574/5; fax: 5371576; Telegram:UNIVVET

E mail:drpabha@tanuvas.com tanuvas@md2.vsnl.net.in; Website:www.tanuvas.com

Vice-Chancellor : Dr. R. Prabhaharan

Tamil Nadu Veterinary and Animal Sciences University is first of its kind in India and was set up by the government of Tamil Nadu by an act of the State Assembly. The university comprises of Madras Veterinary College, Fisheries College and Research Institute, Tuticorn, Veterinary College and Research Institute, Namakkal. The university is set up for the advancement of learning and prosecution of research in veterinary and animals sciences and fisheries and to undertake the extension of such sciences to rural people in cooperation with government departments concerned and various agencies, to impart education in different branches of Veterinary and Animal Sciences and Fisheries.

WEST BENGAL UNIVERSITY OF ANIMAL AND FISHERY SCIENCES

37 & 68, Kshudiram Bose Sarani, Belgachia

Calcutta-700037 (W.B.)

Tel: (033)5565021; Gram:VETUNIV;FAX:033-5571986

Year of Establishment : 2nd January 1995

Vice-Chancellor : Dr. A.K. Bhattacharya

Bengal veterinary college was established in 1893 at belgachia under Calcutta University and was later transferred to Mohanpur, Nadia in 1974 under the Bidhan Chandra Krishi Vishwvidyalaya. In 1995, it was again shifted to Belgachia as West Bengal University of Animal and Fishry Sciences. The university has three faculties viz:

1. Faculty of Veterinary and Animal Sciences Campus; (a) Mohanpur (Nadia) (b) Belgachia (Calcutta)
2. Faculty of Dairy Technology Campus Mohanpur (Nadia)
3. Faculty of Fishery Sciences Campus Kalyani (Nadia)

Chapter - 10

VETERINARY COLLEGES

One who looks retrospectively into the history of veteriinary education, a modest begining of veterinary education may be said to have been made in 1862 with the establishment of an army veterinary school in Pune. The first civil veterinary school was started in Babugarh in district Uttar Pradesh where now at present an army equine stud farm exists. The level of training imparted by these schools was of low standard. Further due to frequent occurrence of famines and cattle plagues several commissions were appointed to look into the control of plagues. On the recommendation of these commissions, a civil veterinary department was established in 1881. Hence, the scientific and rational approach for producing qualified veterinarians was felt by the Britishers who started the first veterinary college at Lahore in 1882 and later at Bombay in 1886, Calcutta in 1892 and Madras in 1903. These institutions started producing trained veterinarians and awarded Diploma every year to successful candidates adopting the course programme developed by Royal College of Veterinary Surgeons, London. These diplomas were called **Graduate of Veterinary College (GVC)**. Teaching of GVC continued for several years. The Bombay and Patna offered graduates of GBVC, while Bengal Veterinary College, Calcutta awarded diploma entitiled **"Graduate of Veterinary Science** and Madras offered graduate of **Madras Veterinary College (GMVC)**. It was felt on the basis of services rendered by these trained veterinarians that they do not meet the required level of skill and knowledge. The Royal Commission of Agriculture in 1928 recommended a four fold increase in the employment of

Veterinary Assistant Surgeons to meet the demand for curing and controlling of diseases. They also suggested that higher education in veterinary science be developed in India on similar lines to that of the Royal College of Veterinary Surgeons in England. As such, the veterinary education should be converted to a degree course offering a BVSc degree. **Bachelor of Veterinary Science (BVSc)** was started for the first time at Madras Veterinary College in 1936 with the affiliation of this college with the university of Madras. With the dawn of independence of India in 1947, a number of veterinary colleges were added. In between 1946 and 1948 five more veterinary colleges were established at Hyderabad, Mathura, Jabalpur, Guwahati and Hisar. Five more colleges were established during the year 1949 and 1956 each at Rajasthan, Orissa, Andhra Pradesh, Madhya Pradesh and Trichur.

One the recommendation of the Indo-American team on Agricultural Education in 1980 and on the lines of Land Grant colleges in the United States, Agricultural Universities were established in 1960. First such university with a veterinary college was opened at Pantnagar in Uatter Pradesh. Within a decade and half, 31 agricultural universities were established. By 1977, all veterinary colleges became affiliated with these universities and became a constituent college of agricultual university. There are now 32 veterinary colleges which are affiliated to 21 State Agricultural Universities (SAU's). Majority of these colleges offer graduate (BVSc), post-graduate (MVSc) and doctorate (PhD) degrees. The role played by Indian Veterinary Research Institute (IVRI) needs a special mention so far as the post-graduate education is concerned. IVRI had post-graduate teaching and training as its integral part from the very early days of its inception and has provided facilities for postgraduate education for scholars from within and outside the country. As early as 1900, training was imparted to field veterinarians in general principle of therapeutics, and to civil and army personnel in comparative pathology, bacteriology and microbiology. These were later replaced by a number of refresher courses for personaale in veterinary profession, IVRI being the National Institute also awarded "Associateship of IVRI" since 1943 to veterinary graduates and this Associateship was taken equivalent to MVSc or MSc for recruitment to higher posts. National Diploma courses in Animal Husbandry, Preventive Medicine, Poultry Husbandry, Animal reproduction, Biological Products and Equine Husbandry were subsequently introduced. With the establishment of post-graduate college of Animal Science in 1958 at IVRI, it could be made possible for the institute to produce post-graduate veterinarians. IVRI has now got the status of a Deemed University from 1983 and is now awarding MVSc and PhD in 22 disciplines of veterinary sciences. In 1950, a post-graduate centre for Veterinary Science was created by the University of Madras at Madras Veterinary College. Creation of a separate university for veterinary and animal sciences in Tamil Nadu was a further step to strengthen the veterinary education.

Owing to a variation in the entrance qualification, duration of the courses curricula and syllabi, evaluation methods and basic infrastructure facilities for teaching, the overall effects of these factors is concerned with the Indian Veterinary degree. The regulation 1933 (minimum standards of veterinary education) laid down by the Veterinary Council of India under the Indian Veterinary Council Act 1984 would now regulate the standards of veterinary education all over the country.

PRIVATE VETERINARY COLLEGE

It is interesting to mention about a private veterinary college namely **"Bhartiya Veterinary College"** which was probably started in 1984 at Bangalore.

Bhartiya Veterinary College

6th Milestone, Kanakapura, J.P. Nagar

Bangalore-560 078

Name of the Dean : Dr. V. G. Patil Kulkarni

Unfortunately, detailed information could not be made available and this college does not exist. However, its logo is reproduced below:

Bharatiya Veterinary College

(A premier Institute to serve people grow with veterinary profession)
6th Milestone, Kanakapur, Road, J.P. Nagar, Bangalore-560 078. India.

Veterinary Colleges (Consolidated List)

Sl.No.	Name of College	Place	Year of Establishment
1.	Bombay Veterinary College	Bombay	1886
2.	Faculty of Veterinary Science	Calcutta	1892
3.	Madras Veterinary College	Chennai	1903
4.	Bihar Veterinary College	Patna	1927
5.	College of Veterinary Science Rajendranagar	Hyderabad	1946
6.	College of Veterinary Sci & AH	Mathura	1947
7.	College of Veterinary Sci & AH	Hisar	1948
8.	College of Veterinary Sci & AH	Jabalpur	1948
9.	College of Veterinary Sci & AH	Guwahati	1948
10.	College of Veterinary Science	Bikaner	1954
11.	College of Veterinary Sci & AH	Bhubneswar	1955
12.	College of Veterinary Sci & AH	Thrissur	1955
13.	College of Veterinary Science	Triupati	1957
14.	Veterinary College	Bangalore	1958
15.	College of Veterinary Sci & AH	Mhow	1958
16.	Nagpur Veterinary College	Nagpur	1958
17.	College of Veterinary Science	Pantnagar	1960
18.	Ranchi Veterinary College	Ranchi	1961
19.	College of Veterinary Sci & AH	Anand	1964
20.	College of Veterinary Science	Ludhiana	1969
21.	College of Veterinary Sci & AH	Parbhani	1972
22.	College of Veterinary Sci & AH	S.K. Nagar	1981
23.	Faculty of Veterinary Science	Srinagar	1984
24.	College of Veterinary Science	Bidar	1984
25.	College of Veterinary Science	Durg	1985
26.	Veterinary College & Research Institute	Namakkal	1985
27.	College of Veterinary Science	Palampur	1986
28.	College of Veterinary Science P.O. Azad, Assam	North Lakhimpur	1987
29.	College of Veterinary Science and Animal Science	Udgir	1987
30.	K.N.P. College of Veterinary Science	Shirval	1988
31.	College of Veterinary Science	Faizabad	1993
32.	Rajiv Gandhi College of Veterinary & Animal Science	Pondicherry	1994
33.	College of Veterinary Science	Mizoram	1998

1. BOMBAY VETERINARY COLLEGE

PAREL, MUMBAI-400012 (M.S.)

Tel: 022-4131180; 4132792; 4130162; Fax: 4130162

Year of Establishment	: 2 August 1886
Affiliation	: Konkan Krishi Vidyapeeth Dapoli Dist : Ratnagiri-415712
Recognition	: Veterinary Council of India
Name of the Dean	: Dr. S. Jagdish
Degree offered	: BVSc&AH, MVSc, PhD

Historical milestones

1. First and original work on South African Horse Sickness, Mucosal disease complex, Gumboro disease and adenovirus infection of poultry in India etc.
2. Extraction of insulin and heparin from buffalo pancreas and lungs respectively.
3. Studies on immunoglobulin in animals, parasitic immunity, immunity to cancer etc.
4. Comparative oncology
5. Zoonotic diseases viz: trichellosis, cysticercosis, rabies, brucellosis, tuberculosis, salmonellosis.
6. Immunological tests for detection of meat adulteration and meat speciation.
7. Establishment of microbiological standards for meat and meat products.
8. Deep freezing of semen and post-partum anoestrus condition
9. Utilization of non-conventional items in animal feeds
10. Chromosomal and genetic studies on cross bred cattle
11. Dialysis, transfusion studies, anorexia, skin diseases in animals
12. Quail husbandry
13. Innovative surgical procedures
14. Important animal diseases and pests like Rinderpest, Canine influenza, canine bordetella, parvovirus, tapeworms, ticks, coccidiosis etc.

2. FACULTY OF VETERINARY AND ANIMAL SCIENCES

[Erstwhile Bengal Veterinary College, Calcutta-37]

37, Kshudiram Bose Sarani, Belgachia, Calcutta-700 037

Tel: 556-5021; Fax: 5571986; Gram:VETUNIV

Year of establishment	:	1892
Affiliation	:	West Bengal University of Animal and Fishery Science
Recognition	:	Veterinary Council of India
Name of the Dean	:	Dr. K. B. Das Bhowmik
Degrees Offered	:	BVSc&AH, MVSc, PhD

3. MADRAS VETERINARY COLLEGE

CHENNAI-600 007

Tel: 044-581506/Ext.227, Direct 562787; Fax : 044-562787;
Telex : 041-5049 MVC IN; Gram:UNIVET

Year of establishment	:	1903
Affiliation	:	Tamil Nadu Veterinary and Animal Sciences University
Recognition	:	Veterinary Council of India
Name of the Dean	:	Dr. R. Kadirvel
Degree/Diploma Offered	:	BVSc,MVSc, PhD, Diploma

Historical events: The Tamil Nadu Veterinary and Animal Sciences University started as an Agricultural School at Sadipet, Madras in 1876, offering Diploma and Certificate courses in the field of Veterinary and Animal Sciences. The school attained the status of a college in 1903. On the recommendation of the Indo-Americal team of Agricultural Research and Education this college was upgraded as a Southern Regional Centre of Post Graduate Education and Research in 1958. Some of informations about this college have been covered under the heading of universities.

4. BIHAR VETERINARY COLLEGE, PATNA

P.O. Patna-800024 Tel: (O) 222231

Year of establishment	:	1927

Affiliation : Rajendra Agricultural University, Bihar, Pusa, Samastipur
Recognition : Veterinary Council of India
Name of the Principal : Dr. P. S. Srivastava
Degree/Diploma Offered : BVSc&AH, MVSc, PhD, Diploma

Historical events: The college was established in the British regime and the foundation stone was laid by Sir Henry Wheeler, the then Governor of Bihar and Orissa in 1927. Initially, the college offered a three years diploma programme called GBVC. The first batch of GBVC diploma holders passed out in 1933. This diploma was upgraded to a four year degree course (BVSc & AH) and the first degree holders passed out in 1954. Post-graduate courses (MVSc) were started in 1960 which was followed by doctorate programme (PhD) and the first PhD student passed out in 1969. Initially, the college was under the control of State Animal Husbandry Department, later in 1970 with the inception of Rajendra Agricultural University, the college was transferred to it.

5. COLLEGE OF VETERINARY SCIENCE

Rajendranagar, Hyderabad-560030 (Andhra Pradesh)

Year of establishment : 1946
Affiliation : Andhra Pradesh Agricultural University, Hyderabad-500030 (AP)
Recognition : Veterinary Council of India
Name of the Principal : Dr. B. Yadgiri
Degrees Offered : BVSc & AH, MVSc, PhD

6. COLLEGE OF VETERINARY SCIENCE & ANIMAL HUSBANDRY

Mathura-201 002 (UP)

Year of establishment : 1947
Affiliation : C. S. Azad University of Agriculture & Technology Kanpur (UP)
Recognition : Veterinary Council of India
Name of the Dean : Dr. M. P. Singh
Degrees Offered : BVSc & AH, MVSc, PhD

7. COLLEGE OF VETERINARY SCIENCE

Hisar-125 004 (Haryana)

Tel:01662-37192; Fax:34952; Gram: VETCOL, AGRIVERSITY

Year of establishment : 1948

Affiliation : Chaudhary Charan Singh Haryana Agricultural University, Hisar

Recognition : Veterinary Council of India

Name of the Dean : Dr. R. D. Sharma

Degree Offered : BVSc & AH, MVSc, PhD, Diploma (VLDA)

History: The history of this college dates back to the year 1882 when the first veterinary school was established in India at Lahore, now in Pakistan. This was subsequently upgraded as a college. After the partition of India in 1947, with the help of staff of the Lahore college who had migrated to India, the Punjab Government set up a camp Veterinary College at Hisar on 15th February 1948. It was affiliated to East Punjab University, Solan for the award of BVSc degree. On 2nd October 1955 the foundation stone of this college buidling was laid down. With the formation of Punjab Agricultural University in 1967, this college was transferred to this university and is now a constituent college of Chaudhary Charan Singh Haryana Agricultural University.

8. COLLEGE OF VETERINARY SCIENCE

South Civil Lines, Jabalpur-482 001 (M.P.)

Tel: 321302 Telegram : VETCOL

Year of establishment : 1948

Affiliation : Jawahar Lal Nehru Krishi Vishwavidyalaya, Jabalpur

Recognition : Veterinary Council of India

Name of the Dean : Dr. K. N. P. Rao

Degrees Offered : BVSc & AH, MVSc & AH, PhD

9. COLLEGE OF VETERINARY SCIENCE

Khanapara, Guwahati-781022 (Assam)

Year of establishment	: 1948
Affiliation	: Assam Agricultural University
Recognition	: Veterinary Council of India
Name of the Dean	: Dr. Dharmeshwar Das
Degrees offered	: BVSc & AH, MVSc, PhD

10. COLLEGE OF VETERINARY AND ANIMAL SCIENCES

Bikaner-334 001 (Rajasthan)

Tel: (O) 543419; : Gram	: RAJVETCOL
Year of establishment	: 1954
Recognition	: Veterinary Council of India
Affiliation	: Rajasthan Agricultural University, Bikaner
Name of the Dean	: Dr. S. S. Sharma
Degrees offered	: BVSc &AH, MVSc, PhD

11. COLLEGE OF VETERINARY SCIENCE AND ANIMAL HUSBANDRY

Bhubneswar-751 003; Gram	: Agritech
Year of establishment	: 1955
Affiliation	: Orissa University of Agriculture and Technology
Recognition	: Veterinary Council of India
Name of the Dean	: Dr. S. C. Mishra
Degrees Offered	: BVSc & AH, MVSc, PhD

12. COLLEGE OF VETERINARY AND ANIMAL SCIENCES

Mannuthy, Thrissur, Kerala-680 651 (Karnataka)

Tel:0487-370451; Fax No. 370019; Telex: 0887 266 KAU IN;

E-mail:vet@Kauren.nic.in

Year of establishment : 1955

Affiliation : Kerala Agricultural University

Recognition : Veterinary Council of India

Name of the Dean : Dr. S. Sulochana

Degrees Offered : BVSc, MVSc, PhD

Milestones: Centre of Advanced Studies in Poultry Science and Animal Husbandry and Genetics; Centre of Excellence in Veterinary Pathology

13. COLLEGE OF VETERINARY SCIENCE

Tirupati-517502; Dist: Chitoor (A.P.)

Tel:08574, 28155; Fax:27932. 27499, 25211

Year of establishment : 1958

Affiliation : Acharya N. G. Ranga Agricultural University

Recognition : Veterinary Council of India

Name of the Dean : Dr. Md. Hafeez

Degrees offered : BVSc & AH, MVSc & AH, Diploma

14. VETERINARY COLLEGE

Hebbal, Bangalore-56 0024 (Karnataka)

Tel: (O) 3410509, 3411483, Telex:0845-8393-USAK-IN; Fax:080-3410509; Gram:UNIVGRIS

Year of establishment : 1958

Affiliation : University of Agricultural Sciences, Hebbal, Bangalore

Recognition : Veterinary Council of India

Director of Instructions : Dr. S. Abdul Rahman

Degrees Offered : BVSc, MVSc, PhD

15. COLLEGE OF VETERINARY SCIENCE & ANIMAL HUSBANDRY

Rasalpura, Mhow (M.P.)

Tel: (O) 73622

Year of establishment : 1958
Affiliation : Jawahar Lal Nehru Vishwavidyalaya Jabalpur
Recognition : Veterinary Council of India
Name of the Dean : Dr. G. P. Tiwari
Degrees Offered : BVSc &AH, MVSc & AH, Diploma

16. NAGPUR VETERINARY COLLEGE

Seminary Hills, Nagpur-444 006 (M.S.) Tel: 531259, 352883
High Land Drive
Year of establishment : 1958
Affiliation : Dr. Panjabrao Deshmukh Krishi Vidyapeeth, Akola
Recognition : Veterinary Council of India
Name of the Dean : Dr. S. D. Harne
Degrees offered : BVSc &AH, MVSc & AH, MVSc

17. COLLEGE OF VETERINARY SCIENCE

Pantnagar-263 145 (UP)
Tel:05948-33347; Fax No:33473; Gram:AGRIVERSITY
Year of establishment : 1960
Affiliation : G. B. Pant University of Agriculture & Technology
Recognition : Veterinary Council of India
Name of the Dean : Dr. Har Pal Singh
Degree Offered : BVSc &AH, MVSc, PhD

18. COLLEGE OF VETERINARY SCIENCE & ANIMAL HUSBANDRY

Kanke, Ranchi-8340 07 (Bihar)
Tel: (O)0651-455324; Gram: VETCOL
Year of establishment : 1961
Affiliation : Birsa Agricultural University

Recognition : Veterinary Council of India
Name of the Dean : Dr. K.P. Yadav
Degree Offered : BVSc &AH, MVSc, PhD
Diploma in Animal Husbandry
Diploma in Poultry Husbandry
Diploma in Swine Husbandry

19. COLLEGE OF VETERINARY SCIENCE & ANIMAL HUSBANDRY

Nr. Jagnath Temple, Ananad, Dist: Kheda
Gujarat State-388001
Tel: (O)o2692-41486; Gram-GUJVET; Fax:41520, 41270
Year of establishment : 1964
Affiliation : Gujarat Agricultural University
Recognition : Veterinary Council of India
Name of the Dean : Dr. Y. G. Dugwekar
Degree offered : BVSc & AH, MVSc, PhD

20. COLLEGE OF VETERINARY SCIENCE

Ludhiana-141 004
Tel: 400822, 401960/210; Fax:400945
Year of establishment : 1969
Affiliation : Punjab Agricultural University
Recognition : Veterinary Council of India
Name of the Dean : Dr. J.S. Dhillon
Degree offered : BVSc &AH, MVSc, PhD

Two departments of the college have been recognised as ICAR Centres of Advanced Studies.

1. ICAR Centre for Advanced Studies in Veterinary Surgery and Radiology
2. ICAR Centre for Advanced Studies in Veterinary Gyaenacology and Obstetrics

21. COLLEGE OF VETERINARY SCIENCE & ANIMAL SCIENCES

Parbhani-431 402 (M.S.)

Tel: 23801-23805, 7&8 Ext. 424; Fax:02452-23582

Year of establishment	: 1972
Affiliation	: Marathwada Agricultural University
Recognition	: Veterinary Council of India
Name of Associate Dean & Principal	: Dr. K.S. Deshpande
Degree offered	: BVSc & AH, MVSc. PhD

22. COLLEGE OF VETERINARY SCIENCE & ANIMAL HUSBANDRY

Sardar Krushinagar-385506 Dist: Banaskantha (Gujarat)

Tel: (O) 02748-77139; Fax:77009

Year of establishment	: 1984
Affiliation	: Gujarat Agricultural University
Recognition	: Veterinary Council of India
Name of the Principal	: Dr. P. L. Kaul
Degree/Certificate offered	: BVSc & AH, MVSc, PhD, Certificate Course of Livetsock Inspectors

23. FACULTY OF VETERINARY SCIENCE & ANIMAL HUSBANDRY

Shuhama (Alusteng), Post Box. 135, Srinagar-Kashmir

Year of establishment	: 1984
Affiliation	: S. K. University of Agricultural Science & Technology (SKUAST)
Recognition	: Veterinary Council of India
Name of Prof. Incharge Academics	: Dr. Shabur Ahmed Mir and Administration
Degree Offered	: BVSc & AH, MVSc

24. VETERINARY COLLEGE

Post Box No.6, Bidar-585 401, Karnataka

Tel: (O) 0842-26149, (R) 26809

Year of establishment	:	1984-85
Affiliation	:	University of Agricultural Sciences, Krishinagar Dharward-580 005
Recognition	:	Veterinary Council of India
Name of the Dean	:	Dr. P. Basavaiah
Degree Offered	:	BVSc & AH, MVSc (in some subjects)

25. COLLEGE OF VETERINARY SCIENCE & ANIMALS HUSBANDRY

Post Box No.6, Anjora, Durg-491001 (M.P.)

Tel: (O)0788-322298 Fax:323215

Year of establishment	:	1985
Affiliation	:	Indira Gandhi Agricultural University, Raipur (M.P.)
Recognition	:	Veterinary Council of India
Name of the Dean	:	Dr. B.C. Gurung
Degree offered	:	BVSc, MVSc

26. VETERINARY COLLEGE AND RESEARCH INSTITUTE

Namakkal-637 001, Rajaji District (TN)

Tel : 66491, 66492, 66493, 66469 Fax No. 23602

Year of establishment	:	1985
Affiliation	:	Tamil Nadu Veterinary and Animal Sciences University Chennai-600 007
Recognition	:	Veterinary Council of India
Name of the Dean	:	Dr. P. Sadasivam
Degree offered	:	BVSc, MVSc, PhD

27. COLLEGE OF VETERINARY & ANIMAL SCIENCES

Palampur, Distt: Kangra (Himachal Pradesh)-176062

Tel : 30327, 30608, Fax : 01894-30511 Gram : VETCOL

Year of establishment : 1986

Affiliation : Himachal Pradesh Krishi Vishvavidyalaya, Palampur

Recognition : Veterinary Council of India

Name of the Dean : Dr. R. Katoch

Degrees offered : BVSc & AH, MVSc, PhD

28. LAKHIMPUR COLLEGE OF VETERINARY SCIENCES

Azad, North Lakhimpur-787 001 (Assam)

Tel : (O) 03752-22670

Year of establishment : 1987-88

Affiliation : Assam Agricultural University

Recognition : Veterinary Council of India

Name of the Dean : Dr. Dharmeswar Das

Degree offered : BVSc & AH

29. COLLEGE OF VETERINARY SCIENCE & ANIMAL SCIENCES

Udgir, Dist: Lature

Tel: (O) 02385-52630 (R) 52836

Year of establishment : 1987

Affiliation : Marathwada Agricultural University, Parbhani

Recognition : Veterinary Council of India

Name of the Dean : Dr. M. A. Gaffar

Degree offered : BVSc & AH

Milestone : The college has developed Deoni breed of cattle of Marthwada region

30. KRANTISINH NANA PATIL COLLEGE OF VETERINARY SCIENCES

Shrival-412 801, Tal: Khandala, Dist: Satara (M.S.)

Year of establishment : 1988

Affiliation : Mahatama Phule Krishi Vidyapeeth Rahuri-413 722 Dist. : Ahmednagar (MS)

Recognition : Veterinary Council of India
Name of the Associate Dean: Dr. A. K. Srivastava
Degree offered : BVSc & AH

31. COLLEGE OF VETERINARY SCIENCE & ANIMAL HUSBANDRY

Narendra Nagar, P.O. Kumar Ganj, Faizabad-224 229 (UP)
Tel: 05270- 62078

Year of establishment : 1993
Affiliation : Narendra Dev University of Agriculture & Technology, Faizabad
Name of the Dean : Dr. S.K. Bhadula
Degree offered : BVSc &AH

32. RAJIV GANDHI COLLEGE OF VETERINARY & ANIMAL SCIENCES

Kurumbapet, Pondicherry-605 009
Tel :(O)0413-71671, 72005 (R), 51961; Fax:72005

Year of establishment : 1994 (Autonomous college)
Affiliation : Pondicherry (Central) University
Recognition : Veterinary Council of India
Name of the Dean : Dr. G. Butchaiah
Degree offered : BVSc & AH

33. COLLEGE OF VETERINARY SCIENCES & ANIMAL HUSBANDRY

Selesih, Aizawl, Mizoram
Tel: 0398-344713, 61324

Year of establishment : 1998
Affiliation : Central Agricultural University Imphal, Manipur
Recogntion : Yet to receive
Name of the Dean : Dr. R. N. Singh, OSD/Dean
Degree offered : BVSc & AH

Chapter - 11

VETERINARY ASSOCIATIONS

There are atleast three types of organisations involved in the development and progress of veterinary profession. They include universities and their colleges which train veterinarians, statutory bodies empowered by government and the professional societies which may be international, national or local. In India in 1919, when there was no agency with specific purpose for co-ordinating work on agriculture and animal husbandry in different provinces and bringing them in line with the policy of Central Government. This promotion and coordination of animal husbandry work was managed with the help of the agricultural advisers to the Government of India, or through conferences of Minsiters and Directors of Agriculture. Most countries have their own professional veterinary society. In our country, there are a number of professional societies which are registered with Society Act 21, 1860. Membership with these societies is optional but veterinarians as per their requirement and choice become member of one or more such societies. In fact, these societies promote the professions's views to the public, government, academic and other institutions.

These societies conduct annual National conferences and symposia sometimes in collaboration with WHO/FAO/UNDP or Indian agencies like ICAR, ICMR, CSIR, DST, NABARD etc. These societies mostly publish journal and/ or a newsletter. They contain subjects both of national and international relevance.

National veterinary associations are usually not only good source of information on the subject or profession in the country but also offer recognition to professionals giving them awards, appreciations or conferring the title of Fellows. In our country, there are mainly two such broad based societies viz: **Indian Veterinary Association** and **Indian Association for the Advancement of Veterinary Research**, which deal with all aspects of veterinary science and animal husbandry. Other societies are either animal species oriented like **Indian Poultry Science Association** or subjects oriented like **Indian Association for the Advancement of Parasitology, Indian Society for Veterinary Surgery, Indian Society of Veterinary Medicine** and so on. The purpose of these societies is to promote the particular veterinary subject.

The societies also develop recommendations which they forward to Ministeries, Universities and other agencies identifying priority areas in research, education and extension. The recommendation of the societies have been helpful in establishment of many laboratories.

Consolidated List of Societies

Sl.	*Name of Society*	*Year of establishment*
1.	Indian Veterinary Association	1924
2.	The Wild Life Preservation Society of India	1958
3.	Indian Poultry Science Association	1965
4.	Indian Association for Animal Production	1969
5.	Indian Society for the Study of Animal Reproduction	1972
6.	Indian Association of Veterinary Pathologists	1974
7.	Indian Society for Veterinary Surgery	1977
8.	Indian Society of Indigenous Veterinary Medicine	1977
9.	Indian Association of Comparative Microbiologists, Immunologists & Specialists in Infectious Diseases	1978
10.	Delhi Veterinary Association	1978
11.	Indian Society for Animal Genetics & Breeding	1978
12.	Society of Toxicology, India	1979
13.	Society of Veterinary Physiologists, Pharmacologists & Biochemists of India	1982
14.	Indian Society for Veterinary Medicine	1981
15.	Indian Association of Veterinary Anatomists	1983
16.	Indian Virological Society	1984

Contd...

Sl.	*Name of Society*	*Year of establishment*
17.	Laboratory Animal Science Association of India	1984
18.	Indian Association of Equine Interests	1984
19.	Society of Animal Physiologists of India	1984
20.	Indian Society for Animal Production & Management	1984
21.	Indian Association for the Advancement of Veterinary Parasitology	1986
22.	Indian Association of Meat Science & Technologies	1986
23.	Indian Lady Veterinary Association	1987
24.	Indian Association of Mycoplasmologists	1988
25.	Indian Society for Veterinary Immunology & Biotechnology	1990
26.	Indian Association for the Advancement of Veterinary Research	1991
27.	Animal Nutrition Association	1993
28.	Indian Association of Deans of Veterinary Colleges	1994
29.	Society for Veterinary Epidemiology & Preventive Medicine	
30.	Society for Human and Animal Mycologists	1995

NATIONAL ASSOCIATIONS

1. INDIAN VETERINARY ASSOCIATION

Historical perspective : The All-India Veterinary Association was founded in 1922 as a result of untiring and selfless efforts of Drs. M.S. Sastry, T.V. Mudaliar, A. Ramalinga Mudaliar and R. Swaminatha Iyer of the erstwhile Madras Presidency and Drs. T. Davis and S.M. Raza Hussain of United Provinces. The name of the association was changed as the Indian Veterinary Association in 1960. The association obtained registration under Society Act 21, 1860 in 1967 and its constitution was revised in 1970. All the States and Union Territories of the Indian Union have formed State Veterinary Association and most of them stand affiliated to the Indian Veterinary association. The Indian Veterinary Association is a founder member of the Commonwealth Veterinary Association established in 1967. The Association was a member of World Veterinary Association since 1970 had to withdraw its membership in 1976 as the World Body insisted on payment of subscription on per capita basis instead of the nominal contribution.

Year of establishment : 1924 (Registered in 1960)

Status	: Registered under Society Act 21,1860
Address	: 123, 7th `B' Main Road IV Block (West) Jayanagar, Bangalore-560 011
Admission eligibility	: Recognised Veterinary Qualification
Member	: All State Associations are affiliated member
President	: Dr.R.S. Sharma
Secretary	: Dr. S. Abdul Rahman
Activities	: Publication of Indian Veterinary Journal, organizing conferences, symposia etc.

2. DELHI VETERINARY ASSOCIATION

WZ-311/A, Nangal Raya, New Delhi-110046

Year of establishment : 1978

Status	: Registered Under Society Act 21,1860 Address : WZ-311/A, Nangal Raya New Delhi-110046
Admission eligibility	: Veterinary Qualification
Number of members	: 316
President	: Dr. Ram Vir Sharma
Secretary	: Dr. J.D. Verma
Activities	: Proposes to publish a quarterly magazine Metro Vet, conducts Seminar and Annual Conferences, Cooperates with other NGOS, Animal Welfare/Treatment Camp.

3. INDIAN ASSOCIATION FOR THE ADVANCEMENT OF VETERINARY RESEARCH

Year of establishment	: 1991
Status of Society	: Registered under Society Act 21,1860
Address	: 363, Bari Bamanpuri, Bareilly-243003(UP)
Admission eligibility	: BVSc &AH

Number of Members : 330
President : Dr. T.N. Jaiswal
Founder Secretary : Dr. Rishendra Verma

Activities : Publication of a journal-The Indian Journal of Veterinary research, organisation of annual conference and symposium, representation to Pay Commission and to other agencies, to keep a liason with government and other such organisations, to undertake work for registration of veterinarians or any such type of help, to make recommendations to government, universities etc on various aspects of veterinary science and education, to keep a link with International veterinary organisations.

4. INDIAN ASSOCIATION OF DEANS OF VETERINARY COLLEGES

Year of establishment : 1994
Status of Society : Registered Under Society Act 21, 1860
Address : Madras Veterinary College
Chennai-600 007
Members : Deans of all Veterinary Colleges
President : Dr. N. Natrajan
Secretary : Dr. S. Shanmugasundaram

Aims and objects: To promote understanding, interaction and exchange of ideas among Heads of Veterinary Colleges of India, to initiate, encourage and support advancement of teaching and research to veterinary institutions, to introduce innovative methods of teaching and conduction of examination, to act as a National Body to represent veterinary education. to cooperate with other professional associations, societies etc both at National and International levels, to institute awards/fellowships/medals, to publish journals, reports etc and to organise conference and symposia.

5. INDIAN ASSOCIATION OF LADY VETERINARIANS*

Year of establishment : 1987
Status of Society : Registered Under Society Act 21,1860

*Present Status of Society uncertain

Address	: 14/115A DDA Flats, Kalkaji, New Delhi -110019
Admission eligibility	: Graduate in Veterinary Science
Number of members	: Not known
President	: Dr. Thankam Mathew
Secretary	: Dr. P. S. Lalitha
Activities	: Publication of Souvenir, Annual Conference

ASSOCIATIONS BASED ON ANIMAL SPECIES

6. THE WILD LIFE PRESERVATION SOCIETY OF INDIA

Year of establishment	: 1958
Status of Society	: Registered Under Society Act 21,1860
Address	: 7, Astley Hall, Dehradun-248 001 (UP)
Number of Members	: 380 (Both Indian & Foreign)
President	: Sri N.D. Bachkheti, IFS (Retd)
Secretary	: Sri I.S. Negi, IFS (Retd)
Activities	: Publication of a quarterly Journal Cheetal, organisation of annual meetings, wildlife excursions, wildlife exhibitions

7. INDIAN POULTRY SCIENCE ASSOCIATION

Year of establishment	: 1965
Status of Society	: Registered under Society Act 21,1860
Address	: Central Avian Research Institute Izatnagar- 243 122 (UP)
Admission eligibility	: Open to persons interested in the objects of the association
Number of Members	: 425
President	: Dr. B. Panda
Secretary	: Dr. S.V.S. Verma
Activities	: Publishes Indian Journal of Poultry Science, Organises Annual Conference and Symposium.

8. LABORATORY ANIMALS SCIENCE ASSOCIATION OF INDIA

Year of establishment	: 1984
Status	: Registered Under Society Act 21, 1860
Address	: National Laboratory Animal Centre Central Drug Research Institute Lucknow-226 001 (UP)
Admission eligibility	: Graduate in Science or Matriculate with 10 years experience in Laboratory Animals
Number of members	: 271
President	: Dr. K. R. Bhardwaj
Secretary	: Dr. D. C. Purohit
Activities	: Publication of a journal- Laboratory Animals India, organisation of symposium

9. THE SOCIETY OF INDIGENOUS VETERINARY MEDICINE

Year of establishment	: 1977
Status	: Registered Under Society Act 21, 1860
Address	: Sharda Nagar, Saharanpur-247001(UP)
Admission eligibility	: Graduate Qualification in Vety. Science or interest in development of Herbal Animal Health
Products President	: Dr. P. B. Kuppuswamy
Secretary	: Dr. Sushil Kumar Agrawal
Activity	: Publishes Indian Journal of Indigenous Medicines

10. INDIAN ASSOCIATION OF EQUINE INTERESTS

Year of establishment	: 1984
Status	: Registered Under Society Act 21, 1860
Address	: C/O Chettinuad Stud & Agricultural Farm Surapet, Orakkadu, P.O. (Via) Sholavaram, Madras-600 067

Admission eligibility : Persons interested in equine research & husbandry

President : Mr. R. Ramakrishnan

Secretary : Dr. T. Rajasekaran

Activity : Publishes a Journal

ASSOCIATIONS BASED ON SUBJECTS

11. THE INDIAN ASSOCIATION FOR ANIMAL PRODUCTION

Year of establishment : 1969

Status of Society : Registered under Society Act 21,1860

Address : E 6, NDSE PII, New Delhi-49

Admission eligibility : Open to all persons actively engaged in scientific, technological/developmental work related to any field of Animal Science

Member : Life members 205

President : Dr. P.N. Bhat

Secretary : Dr. V.K. Taneja

Activities : Publishes The Indian Journal of Animal Production

12. INDIAN SOCIETY FOR THE STUDY OF ANIMAL REPRODUCTION

Year of establishment : 1972

Status of Society : Registered under Society Act 21,1860

Address : Department of Gynaecology & Obstetrics College of Veterinary Sciences G.B. Pant University of Agriculture & Technology, Pantnagar-263 145 (UP)

Admission eligibility : Interest in the field of Animal Reproduction

Members : 1050

President : Dr. A. S. Kaikini

Secretary : Dr. S.N. Maurya

Activities : Publishes Indian Journal of Animal Production, organise annual conference etc.

13. INDIAN ASSOCIATION OF VETERINARY PATHOLOGISTS

Year of establishment : 1974

Status of Society : Registered Under Society Act 21,1860

Address : Division of Pathology
Indian Veterinary Research Institute
Izatnagar-243 122 (UP)

Admission eligibility : Specialization in Veterinary Pathology

Number of Members : 417

President : Dr. J.L. Vegad

Secretary : Dr. R.N.S. Gowda

Activities : Publication of a journal- Indian Journal of Veterinary Pathology, Organisation of Annual Conference and Symposium.

14. INDIAN SOCIETY FOR VETERINARY SURGERY

Year of establishment : 1977

Status : Registered Under Society Act 21, 1860

Address : Dept. of Surgery & Radiology
College of Veterinary Science
Hisar-125 004 (Haryana)

Admission eligibility : Veterinary/medical graduate

Number of members : 740

President : Prof. J. M. Nigam

Secretary : Prof. A. P. Singh

Activities : Publication of Journal, Annual Conferences

15. THE SOCIETY OF INDIGENOUS VETERINARY MEDICINE

Year of establishment : 1977

Status : Registered under Society Act, 21, 1860

Address : The Society of Indigenous Vety Medicines, Sharda Nagar
Saharanpur-247001 (UP)

Admission eligibility : Graduate in Veterinary Science or interest in development of Herbal Animal Health Products

Number of members : 215

President : Dr. P. B. Kuppuswamy

Secretary : Shri Sushil Kumar Agrawal

Activities : Publication of Indian Journal of Indigenous Medicines.

16. INDIAN ASSOCIATION OF COMPARATIVE MICROBIOLOGY, IMMUNOLOGY & SPECIALISTS IN INFECTIOUS DISEASES

Year of establishment : 1978

Status : Registered Under Society Act 21, 1860

Address : C/O Division of Avian Disease
Indian Veterinary Research Institute
Izatnagar-243 122 (UP)

Number of members : 300 (Approx.)

President : Dr. K. K. Baxi

Secretary : Dr. P. C. Harbola

Activities : Publication of Journal, Anuual Conferences

17. INDIAN SOCIETY FOR ANIMAL GENETICS & BREEDING

Year of establishment : 1978

Status : Registered Under Society Act 21, 1860

Address : Livestock Economics Division IVRI,
Izatnagar-243 122 (UP)

President : Dr. P. N. Bhat

Secretary : Dr. V. K. Taneja

Activities : Publication of a Journal, Annual Conferences

18. SOCIETY OF TOXICOLOGY, INDIA

Year of establishment : 1979

Status : Registered Under Society Act 21, 1860

Address : Division of Pharmacology & Toxicology IVRI, Izatnagar-243 122 (UP)

Admission eligibility : MSc with experience in Toxicology

Number of members : 400

President : Dr. S. K. Tandon

Secretary : Dr. M. Athar

Activities : To publish a journal, annual conference

19. INDIAN SOCIETY FOR VETERINARY MEDICINE

Year of establishment : 1981

Status of Society : Registered Under Society Act 21,1860

Address : Department of Veterinary Medicine Punjab Agricultural University Ludhiana-141004

Admission eligibility : Graduate of Veterinary Science

Number of Members : 500

President : Dr. S.K. Dwivedi

Secretary : Dr. S.S. Randhawa

Activities : Publication of a journal- The Indian Journal of Veterinary Medicine, Organisation of Annual Conference and Symposium

20. SOCIETY OF VETERINARY PHYSIOLOGISTS, PHARMACOLOGISTS AND BIOCHEMISTS OF INDIA

Year of establishment	:	1982
Status of Society	:	Registered Under Society Act 21,1860
Address	:	Division of Physiology & Climatology Indian Veterinary Research Institute Izatnagar-243 122 (UP)
Admission eligibility	:	Not mentioned
Number of Members	:	Not known
President	:	Dr. J.N Panda
Secretary	:	Dr. P.C. Sanwal
Activities	:	Publication of a journal-Journal of Veterinary Physiology & Allied Sciences

21. INDIAN ASSOCIATION OF VETERINARY ANATOMISTS

Year of establishment	:	1983
Status of Society	:	Registered under Society Act 21,1860
Address	:	Nagpur Veterinary College Nagpur-44006 (M.S.)
Admission eligibility	:	A degree or diploma in Vety. Science A postgraduate degree or diploma in any branch of Vety. Anatomy from statutory body under Govt.
Member	:	150
President	:	Dr. R. P. Saigal
Secretary	:	Dr. V. R. Bhamburkar
Activities	:	Publication of Indian Journal of Veterinary Anatomy

22. INDIAN VIROLOGICAL SOCIETY

Year of establishment	:	1984
Status of Society	:	Registered under Society Act 21,1860
Address	:	CCS Haryana Agricultural University Hisar-125 004 (Haryana)

Admission eligibility : Any graduate doing research in Virology
Member : 220
President : Dr. M.P. Yadav
Secretary : Dr. R.N. Srivastava
Activities : Publication of Indian Journal of Virology, organisation of Annual Conference & Symposia

23. SOCIETY OF ANIMAL PHYSIOLOGISTS OF INDIA

Year of establishment : 1984
Status of Society : Registered Under Society Act 21,1860
Address : National Institute of Animal Nutrition & Physiology
Adugodi, Bangalore-560030
Number of Members : Approx. 300
President : Dr. Kiran Singh
Secretary : Dr. Khub Singh
Activities : Publication of journal- Indian Journal of Animal Physiology, organisation of symposium

24. INDIAN SOCIETY FOR ANIMAL PRODUCTION & MANAGEMENT

Year of establishment : 1984
Status : Registered Under Society Act 21,1860
Address : Department of Animal Production and Management, OUAT,
Bhubneswar-751 003
Number of members : 200(Approx.)
President : Dr. M. Mishra
Secretary : Dr. A. Mohanty
Activity : Publication of a journal

25. INDIAN ASSOCIATION FOR THE ADVANCEMENT OF VETERINARY PARASITOLOGY

Year of establishment : 1986
Status of Society : Registered under Society Act, 21,1860
Address : Department of Parasitology
Bihar Veterinary College, Patna-14
Admission eligibility : Graduate in Science
Members : 267
President : Col (Dr) G.S.C. Rangarao
Secretary : Dr. R.V.N. Srivastava
Activities : Publication of a journal- Journal of Veterinary Parasitology, organisation of conference and symposium

26. INDIAN ASSOCIATION OF MEAT SCIENTISTS & TECHNOLOGISTS*

Year of establishment : 1986
Status of Society : Registered under Society Act 21,1860
Address : Division of Livestock Products Technology, IVRI, Izatnagar-243 122 (UP)
Admission eligibility : Graduate/Diploma holders in meat science
Life Members : 25
President : Dr. A.K. Chatterji
Founder Secretary : Dr. Nagendra Sharma
Activities : Publication of Indian J. Meat Science & Technology, organisation of symposia.

*** Presently the association's working uncertain**

27. INDIAN ASSOCIATION OF MYCOPLASMOLOGISTS

Year of establishment : 1988
Status : Registered Under Society Act 21, 1860
Address : 227-P sector 15-A, Hisar
Admission eligibility : Any person interested in Mycoplasma & related aspects

Number of members : 26 Life Members
President : Dr. D. N. Garg
Secretary : Dr. P. K. Kapoor
Activities : To conduct seminar, workshop, publish JAM News Letter in two years.

28. INDIAN SOCIETY FOR VETERINARY IMMUNOLOGY AND BIOTECHNOLOGY

Year of establishment : 1990
Status of Society : Registered under Society Act 21,1860
Address : Department of Animal Biotechnology Madras Veterinary College, Chennai-7
Admission eligibility : Veterinarians & Non-veterinarians working in Animal Biotechnology & Immunology
Number of members : 273
President : Dr. V.D. Padmanaban
Secretary : Dr. K. Nachimuthu
Activities : Publication of News Letter, organisation of conference and symposium

29. ANIMAL NUTRITION ASSOCIATION

Year of establishment : 1993
Status of Society : Registered under Society Act 21,1860
Address : Division of Animal Nutrition Indian Veterinary Research Institute Izatnagar-243 122 (UP)
: Any reseacher. teacher of Animal
Admission eligibility : Nutrition & allied subjects
Number of Members : 225
President : Dr. N.N. Pathak
Secretary : Dr. D.N. Kamra
Activities : Publication of biannual News Letter, organisation of conference and symposium.

30. SOCIETY FOR VETERINARY EPIDEMIOLOGY & PREVENTIVE MEDICINE

Year of establishment	: 1995
Status of Society	: Registered under society Act 21,1860
Address	: Department of Preventive Medicine Madras Veterinary College Chennai-7 (Tamil Nadu)
Admission eligibility	: Veterinarians in the fields of Veter- inary Preventive Medicine, Vety. Med., Microbiology, Parasitology, Vety. Public Health & Meat Sciences
President	: Dr. R. Manickam
Secretary	: Dr. V.N. Appajirao
Activities	: Organisation of Conference and Symposium

31. SOCIETY FOR INDIAN HUMAN AND ANIMAL MYCOLOGISTS

Year of establishment	: 1995
Status of Society	: Registered Under Society Act 21, 1860
Address	: Department of Biological Science R.D. University, Jabalpur-482 001 (MP)
Secretary	: Prof. S.M. Singh

Chapter - 12

JOURNALS AND OTHER PERIODICALS

We are living in the world what is called "information explosion". A voluminous literature on veterinary and animal sciences existed in ancient India. The Vedas contained repositories of informations of early medicine. In the post-vedic times, Sanskrit literature abounds allusions to veterinary science. Some of the noteworthy examples of this period include Kautilya who in his Arthashastra provided a detailed review on organisation of department of livestock during Chandragupta Maurya's time (322-298 BC). During the period of Kaniska (120-162 AD) a veterinary book was published by an annonymous specialist. In the 13th century AD, the Jain scholar Hamsdeva wrote a natural history of animals called Mriga Pakshi Sastra. Some of the other early books namely Samhita, Brihat, Parasara Samhita, Linga, Purana, Kavi Kalpalata describe about care and treatment of animals.

Grellier (1802) published a book entitled **The Elements of Veterinary Science or The Veterinary Art in India** dealing with the physiology and pathology of the horse in Madras. According to J.R. Hoey (1841) a Veterinary Surgeon in the East India Company's service deplored the lack of veterinary literature in India. Hallen (1871) brought out a publication entitled **More Deadly Forms of Cattle Disease in India"** which gained great popularity. Previous to this, the only publication available to the public was Gilchrist's **Practical Treatise** on treatment of diseases of the elephant etc. In fact veterinary science did not progress rapidly till the issue of the report of the Indian Plague Commission in 1871. A large number of communications from veterinarians, both in H.M.'s and the Company's Army, and from medical men interested in the veterinary work appeared in the pages of The Veterinarian, The Veterinary Record, the Transactions of the Veterinary Medical Association and in Calcutta medical journals. Charles Steel with his associates Fred Smith (Veterinary Surgeon, (12th Lancers) and J.H. Steel (Veterinary Surgeon, Artillery) can be considered the **Father of Modern Journalism in Veterinary Science** for editing **Quarterly Journal of Veterinary Science and Animal Management**, the first journal in 1882 in India which is also claimed to be the first veterinary journal in the world to deal with military veterinary science. These names must be remembered with pride and gratitude by the veterinary profession. This journal made a great impact on the profession not only in India but in all English speaking parts of the world including United-Kingdom.

The journal covered subjects as military campaigns, veterinary education, cruelty to animals, grasses of the Madras Presidency, military veterinary hygiene by Fred Smith and a Materia Medica for India by J.H. Steel. The second issue of the journal contained an article on the Amrat Mahal Cattle Breeding Establishment of Mysore. The journal also supported in 1886 authorities in the establishment of a Civil Veterinary Department. In 1887 Hallen, in his capacity of Honorary Adviser to the Government of India, also contended for a Civil Veterinary Department. The journal again supported his views and highlighted it in an editorial. The publication of the journal continued up to 1890. Steel was the sole editor of the last publication of the journal and died at the beginning of the following year.

After eighteen years of the demise of Steel, another attempt to publish a journal was made in 1905 for veterinary science in India. This journal was called **Journal of Tropical Veterinary Science** and was edited by H.T. Pease, F.S.H., Baldrey and R.E. Montogomery all being members of the Civil Veterinary Department. The early volumes of this journal contained papers on different aspects of surra, animal parasites such as piroplasms and spirochaetes and to some extent helminths. In 1909, the journal covered a wider field and its editorship was taken over by the Inspector General of the Department. This brought misfortune for the journal as the post was abolished and the journal had a natural death and its publication ceased in 1912.

Veterinary profession in India was again left without a high-grade scientific journal for many years.

In 1884, the publication of the Scientific Memoirs by Medical Officers of the Army in India was launched. The series was intended to furnish a convenient medium for the circulation of selected original papers on scientific subjects, which had been the custom to include in the Annual Report of the Sanitary Commissioner with the Government of India. Twelve parts of the **Scientific Memoirs** have been published, the last in 1901 (Cited by B. Franklin, Surgeon- General, I.M.S., Office of the Sanitary Commissioner with the Government of India, Simla, June 30, 1902). In 1900, the **Indian Fowl Farmer's** and **Farmer's Journal** were started. In 1910 the poultry specialists started publication of the journal- **Indian Poultry Gazette**, to publish research in the area of poultry production.

With the wave of intensification of veterinary colleges at graduate and postgraduate levels, veterinarians have realized as early as 1924 that publication of scientific achievements and creation of a common platform to discuss pragmatic problems through seminars and conferences would be inevitable to the veterinary profession. In order to keep pace with ever growing veterinary science and research, a resolution was passed at the Second All India Veterinary Conference held at Lahore in 1923 to start the **"Indian Veterinary Journal (IVJ)"** in English. The earlier failure in publication of the journal in South discouraged veterinarians to accept such a challenge. It seemed to be 'hard nut to crack'. In 1924, Dr. P. Srinivas Rao, a bold veterinarian was entrusted this challenge who edited the IVJ successfully for 31 years. Efforts of Dr. Rao put the IVJ on sound footing with the result that the IVJ is still being regularly published.

Another ecent in veterinary journalism was publication of two new journals namely **Agricultural Journal of India** which was named as **Agriculture and Livestock in India**. This journal included abstracts of research in agriculture and animal sciences. It continued to be published twice a year for nine years. Later, in the year 1940, it was decided to give information in popular English in this periodical and as such it was renamed as **Indian Farming**. Mr. F.M. de Mella was the editor of this popular periodical. In 1945, Dr. Usha Nath Chatterjee, a plant physiologist joined as the Editor of Indian Farming and a new policy was adopted that Indian Farming should highlight current problems of rural development taking into considerations of Indian farmers. Under the patronage of Mr.K.M. Munshi, Minister of Agriculture, in 1951, the Indian Farming took entirely a new shape and size (size of 7.5" x 10" changed to 9" x 11.5"). Mr. M.G. Kamath took over as the Editor of this jorunal in 1954 who further improved the journal. The journal covers three basic sections viz: crop sciences, animal sciences and features e.g. symposia and seminars, advances in farm research, book-reviews and editorial.

"Indian Journal of Veterinary Science and Animal Husbandry" was also started in 1931 under the aegis of Imperial Council of Veterinary Research. The name of this journal was changed to **"Indian Journal of Animal Sciences"** from the year 1969 which publishes articles of veterinary and animal science and is regularly published by the Indian Council of Agricultural Research (ICAR), New Delhi. It is the top most journal of the Council and deals with animal breeding, diseases, physiology, nutrition, dairying, animal production technology and fisheries. It was quarterly till 1966, bimonthly during 1967 and 1968 and is now published monthly since 1969.

After independence, a need of a journal in Hindi to promote scientific farming among the Indian farmers should be started which resulted in the institution of **"Kheti"** in 1948. Mr. Devendrs Satyarthi edited this journal. Since then Kheti is regularly being published by the Indian Council of Agricultural Research. Its basic object was to bridge the gap between the scientist and farmer. Since Mahatma Gandhi had said "India lives in villages", most of rural population can understand scientific matters in Hindi. As such Kheti provides an excellent service for dissemination of knowledge to farmers. Its contents include editorial, question and answers, information on scientific experiments, about new books, news and views. Topics on Pashupalan were included in the publication of Kheti from 1966. Mr. Kuldeep Sharma is its present Chief Editor. The ICAR started a popular journal, **Indian Livestock** in 1963. This was a quarterly. Hindi Pashupalan was merged with kheti.

Management of Journals

The journals are mainly managed with the provisions of a particular scientific society. The journals have Chief Editor, Editor, Associate Editor, Editorial Board and Advisory Board. Some of the name are ornamental. Most of the persons involved with journal publication are tennural office-bearer of the society. The referral system also varies from journal to journal. The refrees in most of the cases are not paid and are expected to help the science by evaluating scientific research papers.

Abstracting of Journals

The journals are abstracted in one or the other abstracting agencies like C.A.B. International, U.K., e.g., Veterinary Bulletin, Index Veterinarius and other CAB abstracting journals; Current Contents, Institute for Information, Philadelphia, USA, INSDOC, New Delhi, India.

Status and Finances of Journals

After 70's and onwards specialization and organised veterinary research resulted into fragmentation of veterinary service into various disciplines. probably, the policy makers would have thought to give full impetus to various animal species and subjects as well as to compete globally with the expanding veterinary science. As a result of which species-wise research institutes were created. Similarly, the subjects in veterinary science were given special consideration and numerous disciplines in the form of individual departments were created in research institutes and college as well. This phenomenon in turn resulted into publication of specialized journal to cater to the needs of specialists and to give more sound footing to progress of individual subjects.

Thus, at present, if one goes through the journal boom, one can find journals on animals species like **Indian Journal of Poultry Science, Journal of Camel Practice and Research, Laboratory Animals India**. Similarly, there are journals which are sibject or a particular discipline oriented like **Journal of Parasitology, Indian Journal of Veterinary Pathology, Indian Journal of Veterinary Surgery, Journal of Meat Science and Technology**.

There are restricted number of journals which cater to needs of all veterinary science and animal husbandry subjects e.g., **Indian Veterinary Journal, Indian Journal of Veterinary Research, Indian Veterinary Medical Journal, Indian Journal of Animal Health**. Some of the journals which have perished include names **Veterinary Research Journal** published College of Veterinary Science and Animal hsubandry, Mathura, **Agra University Journal, Indian Journal of Meat Science and Technology, Indian Poultry Gazette**. Some of the journals are also at the stage of their extinction or they do not have regular periodicity. Probably the farsightedness has also played a vivid role in veterinary journalism and without considering the availability of funds, the journals lost their original periodicity of quarterly or biannual and have obtained a periodicity of biannual or annual respectively.

Most of the journals and magazines are published on letter press. However, few journals like **Indian Journal of Animal Science, Indian Veterinary Journal, Indian Journal of Veterinary Pathology, Indian Journal of Poultry Science, Indian Journal of Veterinary Surgery, Indian Journal of Toxicology** have shifted their performance to off-set printing process. The expenditure becomes almost double of the letter press in the off-set printing thus acting as a constraint for the survival of the journal.

The publication of journals owned by private sectors is in restricted proportion in India. Some of jorunals which are published privately include **International Journal of Animal Science, Journal of Applied Animal Research**. Instead, most of the journals are published as an activity of a particular professional society. And in those cases, survival of a particular society. Most of the journal publication is assisted by respective society funds or the journal publication is assisted by respective society funds or the journals acquire income through library subscriptions, individual subscription, reprint charges and advertisements. The terms and conditions of all the journals for printing of papers are not uniform and vary widely. The Indian Council of Agricultural Research (ICAR) also provide funds to societies as an assistance for publication of the journal thus promoting science. However, the financial assistance to journals by the ICAR is very restricted. Thus, publication of a journal can not necessarily depend on the ICAR grant.

Quality of Production

The quality of journals as such can not be said to be highly satisfactory. This is again due to non-availability of funds with the Society which publishes the journal. There is a general understanding that quality of journal is dependent on the Editor of the journal. But in fact, the quality of the production of a journal depend much on its finances, contributors and subscribers. It is a general tendency to submit high quality papers in journals abroad to get more weightage in career and employment. This is one of the major risk factor for Indian journal. The additional points which need to be added include the fearfulness of authors about the survivability of Indian journal, their periodicity, abstracting and prompt disposal. In the present scenario when the number of journals have increased based on animal species or a particular subject, there is a great crises for the journals to receive good papers. In other words, there is now intraspecific struggle for the survivability among journals. This is in turn has reduced the quality of papers. There are instances wherein a paper is rejected by a journal if it was sent for publishing in any other jorunal.

Another constraint in the process of journal publication is the referral system. The referees have least interest to examine the papers due to their own preoccupations, else the referees retain the papers for a long time thus delay the publication of research data. Sometimes, the referees do not examine the papers meticulously and return the papers in a acusal manner. The referees are not probably paid any honorarium to examine the papers. The authors of the papers also do not take proper care for their submission. They most often do not follow the style of the journal in which they submit their papers. This also causes an unwanted delay in the process. Sometimes delay in transits also play role.

Now the time has come, when the publishers of the journal have to think seriously to compete globally. The history of veterinary journalism tells us that since the inception of first journal in 1882 onwards, there have been a lot of failures in publication. This situation warrants a careful attention.

Magazines and Newspapers

Technical and popular magazines as well as Newspapers in the area of Veterinary Science and Animal Husbandry have tremendously helped in the dissemination of knowledge down to grass rootlevel. In this regard the role of **Indian Farming, Kheti, Dairy Guide, Poultry Guide, Livestock Advisor, Poultry Advisor, The Veterinarian** has been splendid. The newspaper like **Pashudhan, Poultry Reporter, Poultry Flash, Poultry Flame** have significantly added to the dissemination of knowledge and current know-how of Veterinary Science and Animal Husbandry. Publication of some state magazines like **"Prasar Patrika"** by Veterinary College, Mathura, **Indian Farmer's Digest** by G.B. Pant University, Pantnagar, **Haryana Veterinarian** by CCS Haryana Agricultural University, Hisar, **Farmer's Journal, Gosamvardhan** have played a vital role in this regard.

Many veterinary colleges and research institutes publish their own **News Letter** or **Souvenirs** which also contribute knowledge in veterinary scince. Some time the National News papers like Hindu, The Hindustan Times etc publish important discoveries of veterinary research and thus keep the interested readers abreast of the current happenings round the world.

No. 1

(NEW SERIES)

SCIENTIFIC MEMOIRS

BY

OFFICERS OF THE MEDICAL AND SANITARY DEPARTMENTS

OF THE

GOVERNMENT OF INDIA

Standardisation of Calmette's Anti-Venomous Serum with Pure Cobra Venom : The Deterioration of this Serus through Keeping in India

BY

G. Lamb, M.B., Captain, I.M.S., and Wm. Hanna, Esq. M.B., Etc.

(From the Plague Research Laboratory, Bombay)

ISSUED UNDER THE AUTHORITY OF THE GOVERNMENT OF INDIA BY THE SANITARY COMMISSIONER WITH THE GOVERNMENT OF INDIA, SIMLA

THE

QUARTERLY JOURNAL

OF

VETERINARY SCIENCE IN INDIA

AND

ARMY ANIMAL MANAGEMENT

EDITED BY

CHARLES STEEL, F.R.C.V.S., I.V.S., (Bombay Army)

Superintendent Army Veteriany School, Poona.

Assisted by

Fred Smith, V.S., 12th Royal Lancers

John Henry Steel, VS., D.D., Royal Artillery H.S.F.

VOLUME 1., 1883.

Madras :

London :

FASCIMILE OF THE QUARTERLY JOURNAL OF 1883

CONSOLIDATED LIST OF JOURNALS

Sl. No.	Journal Title	Year of Publication
1.	Quarterly Journal of Veterinary Science and Animal Management	1882
2.	Journal of Tropical Veterinary Science	1906
3.	Indian Poultry Gazette	1910
4.	The Indian Veterinary Journal	1924
5.	The Indian Journal of Animal Science	1931
6.	Indian Journal of Dairy Science	1948
7.	Agra University Journal of Research	1952
8.	Indian Journal of Animal Health	1960
9.	The Haryana Veterinarian	1961
10.	The Journal of the Remount & Veterinary Corps	1962
11.	Journal of Research (PAU)	1964
12.	Indian Journal of Poultry Science	1966
13.	Indian Journal of Animal Research	1967
14.	Indian Journal of Animal Production	1970
15.	Journal of Animal & Veterinary Science	1970
16.	The Orissa Veterinary Journal	1970
17.	HAU Journal of Research	1971
18.	Cherion	1972
19.	Indian Journal of Veterinary Pathology	1976
20.	Indian Veterinary Medical Journal	1977
21.	Veterinary Research Journal	1978
22.	The Indian Journal of Animal Genetics and Breeding	1979
23.	Indian Journal of Veterinary Surgery	1980
24.	Indian Journal of Animal Reproduction	1980
25.	Indian Journal of Veterinary Medicine	1981
26.	Journal of Physiology and Allied Sciences	1982
27.	Indian Journal of Animal Nutrition	1984
28.	Centaur	1984
29.	Indian Journal of Virology	1985
30.	Indian Journal of Animal Production and Management	1985
31.	Journal of Applied Animal Research	1986
32.	International Journal of Animal Science	1986

Contd....

Sl. No.	Journal Title	Year of Publication
33.	Journal of Veterinary Parasitology	1987
34.	Laboratory Animals India	1988
35.	Indian Journal of Meat Science and Technology	1988
36.	Indian Journal of Comparative Microbiology Immunology and Infectious Diseases	1988
37.	The Journal of Bombay Veterinary College	1989
38.	Indian Journal of Veterinary Anatomy	1989
39.	The Indian Journal of Veterinary Research	1992
40.	Indian Journal of Toxicology	1992
41.	Indian Journal of Animal Physiology	1992
42.	Journal of Camel Practice and Research	1994
43.	The Indian Journal of Small Ruminants	1995

1. INDIAN POULTRY GAZETTE*

Year of establishment : 1910

Published by : Indian Poultry Club IVRI, Izatnagar

Periodicity : Quarterly

*** Out of Print**

2. THE INDIAN VETERINARY JOURNAL

Year of establishment : 1924

Published by : Indian Veterinary Association

Periodicity : Monthly

Name & address of editor : Dr. V.D. Padmanaban 7, Chamiers Road Chennai-600 035 (Tamil Nadu)

3. INDIAN JOURNAL OF ANIMAL SCIENCE

[Formerly known as Indian Journal of Veterinary Science and Animal Husbandry]

Year of establishment : 1931

Published by : Indian Council of Agricultural Research

Periodicity : Monthly

Name & address of editor : Mrs Aruna T Kumar
Publication & Information Division, Indian Council of Agricultural Research (ICAR) Krishi Anusandhan Bhavan Pusa, New Delhi-110012

4. INDIAN JOURNAL OF DAIRY SCIENCE

Year of establishment : 1948
Published by : Indian Dairy Association
Periodicity : Monthly
Name & address of editor : Dr. A.K. Dodeja
Indian Dairy Association
IDA House, Sector IV R.K. Puram, New Delhi-22

5. AGRA UNIVERSITY JOURNAL OF RESEARCH*

Year of establishment : 1952
Published by : Agra University, Agra
Periodicity : Thrice a year

*** Now out of Print**

6. INDIAN JOURNAL OF ANIMAL HEALTH

Year of establishment : 1960
Published by : West Bengal Veterinary Association
Periodicity : Bi-annual
Name & address of editor : Dr. M.S. Das
68, Belgachia Road
Calcutta-700 037 (W.B.)

7. THE HARYANA VETERINARIAN

[Formerly known as Punjab Veterinarian]

Year of establishment : 1961
Published by : College of Veterinary Science
Hisar-125 004 (Haryana)
Periodicity : Annual

Name & address of editor : Dr. M.U. Kharole
Professor Department of Pathology
College of Veterinary Science
Hisar-125 004 (Haryana)

8. THE JOURNAL OF THE REMOUNT AND VETERINARY CORPS

Year of establishment : 1962
Published by : RVC Centre and School
Periodicity : Quarterly
Name & address of editor : Dr. K. S. Sodhi
Punjab Agricultural University
Ludhiana-141 004 (Punjab)

10. INDIAN JOURNAL OF POULTRY SCIENCE

Year of Publication : 1966
Published by : Indian Poultry Science Association
Periodicity : Quarterly
Name & address of editor : Dr. R.P. Moudgal
Head Division of Avian Physiology & Reproduction Central Avian Research Institute,
Izatnagar-243 122 (UP)

11. INDIAN JOURNAL OF ANIMAL RESEARCH

Year of Publication : 1967
Published by : Agricultural Research Communication Centre, Karnal Periodicity : Bi-annual
Name & address of editor : Dr. D.D. Sharma
Animal Nutrition Division
National Dairy Research Institute
Karnal-132 001 (Haryana)

12. JOURNAL OF ANIMAL AND VETERINARY SCIENCE

Year of establishment : 1970
Published by : University Publication
Periodicity : Bi-annual
Name & address of editor : Dr. K. N. Muraleedharan Nayar
Department of Surgery
College of Veterinary and Animal Sciences, Mannuthy Trichur, Kerala

13. INDIAN JOURNAL OF ANIMAL PRODUCTION

Year of establishment : 1970
Published by : Indian Association for Animal Production
Periodicity : Quarterly
Editor* : Dr. (Mrs) P.P. Bhat

14. THE ORISSA VETERINARY JOURNAL

Year of establishment : 1970
Published by : Orissa Veterinary Association
Periodicity : Quarterly
Name & address of editor : Dr. P. C. Dey
Orissa Veterinary Association
Neelakantha Nagar, Bhubneswar-12

15. HAU JOURNAL OF RESEARCH

Year of establishment : 1971
Published by : University Publication
Periodicity : Quarterly
Name & address of editor : Dr. R. P. Bansal
Directorate of Publications
CCS Haryana Agricultural University, Hisar-125 004

16. CHERION

Year of establishment	: 1972
Published by	: University Publication
Periodicity	: Bi-annual
Name & address editor	: Dr. G. Rajavelu Madras Veterinary College Chennai-600 007 (T.N.)

17. INDIAN JOURNAL OF VETERINARY PATHOLOGY

Year of establishment	: 1976
Published by	: Indian Association of Veterinary Pathologists
Periodicity	: Bi-anual
Name & address of editor	: Dr. M.C. Prasad Division of Pathology Indian Veterinary Research Institute, Izatnagar-243 122 (UP)

18. INDIAN VETERINARY MEDICAL JOURNAL

Year of establishment	: 1977
Published by	: U.P. Veterinary Association
Periodicity	: Quarterly
Name & address of editor	: Dr. J. N. S. Yadav Directorate of Animal Husbandry Badshahbagh, Lucknow-2260 07(UP)

19. VETERINARY RESEARCH JOURNAL*

Year of establishment	: 1978
Published by	: College of Veterinary Science & Animal Husbandry, Mathura
Periodicity	: Bi-annual
Name & address of editor	: Dr. S. S. Mishra Department of Surgery College of Veterinary Science & Animal Husbandry Mathura-(UP)

*** Out of Print**

20. THE INDIAN JOURNAL OF ANIMAL GENETICS & BREEDING

Year of establishment : 1979

Published by : Indian Society of Animal Genetics & Breeding

Name & address of editor : Dr (Mrs) P.P. Bhat

21. INDIAN JOURNAL OF ANIMAL REPRODUCTION

Year of establishment : 1980

Published by : Indian Society for the study of Animal Reproduction

Name & address of editor : Dr. S. R. Pittabiraman, Prof. & Head Department of Clinics Madras Veterinary College, Chennai-600 007 (T.N.)

22. INDIAN JOURNAL OF VETERINARY SURGERY

Year of establishment : 1980

Published by : Indian Society for Veterinary Surgery

Periodicity : Bi-annual

Name & address of editor : Dr. Gajraj Singh
Head, Division of Surgery Indian Veterinary Research Institute, Izatnagar-243 122(UP)

23. INDIAN JOURNAL OF VETERINARY MEDICINE

Year of establishment : 1981

Published by : Indian Society for Veterinary Medicine

Periodicity : Bi-annual

Name & address of editor : Dr. D. Swarup
Senior Scientist, Division of Medicine Indian Veterinary Research Institute, Izatnagar-243122 (U.P.)

24. JOURNAL OF PHYSIOLOGY AND ALLIED SCIENCES

Year of establishment : 1982
Published by : Society of Veterinary Physiologists, Pharmacologists and Biochemists
Periodicity : Bi- annual
Name & address of editor : Dr. P. C. Sanwal
Principal Scientist Division of Physiology & Climatology Indian Veterinary Research Institute, Izatnagar-243 122(UP)

25. INDIAN JORUNAL OF ANIMAL NUTRITION

Year of establishment : 1984
Published by : Animal Nutrition Society of India
Periodicity : Quarterly
Name & address of editor : Dr. K. K. Singhal
Division of Cattle Nutrition National Dairy Research Institute, Karnal

26. CENTAUR

Year of establishment : 1984
Published by : Indian Association of Equine Interests
Periodicity : Bi-annual
Name & address of editor : Dr. C. K. Bhuvana Kumar
C/O Chettinad Stud & Agriculture Farm, Surapet, Orakkadu, P.O.
Via Sholavaram, Chennai-600067

27. INDIAN JOURNAL OF VIROLOGY

Year of establishment : 1985
Published by : Indian Virological Society
Periodicity : Bi-annual
Name & address of editor : Dr. S. M. Paul Khurana
Central Potato Research Institute, Shimla-171 001 (Himachal Pradesh)

28. INDIAN JOURNAL OF ANIMAL PRODUCTION & MANAGEMENT

Year of establishment : 1985
Published by : Indian Society of Animal Production & Management
Name & address of editor : Dr. O. S. Tomer
Division of Cattle Breeding National Dairy Research Institute
Karnal-132 001 (Haryana)

29. JOURNAL OF APPLIED ANIMAL RESEARCH

Year of establishment : 1986
Published by : Garuda Scientific Publications
Periodicity : Quarterly
Name & address of editor : Dr. D.K. Agrawal
151, Janakpuri, P.B. No.6
Izatnagar-243 122 (UP)

30. INTERNATIONAL JOURNAL OF ANIMAL SCIENCE

Year of establishment : 1986
Published by : Nitasha Publication
Periodicity : Bi-annual
Name & address of editor : Mrs Sadhana Jindal
921, Sector 14 Sonepat-131 001 (Haryana)

31. JOURNAL OF VETERINARY PARASITOLOGY

Year of establishment : 1987
Published by : Indian Association for the Advancement of Veterinary Parasitology
Periodicity : Bi-annual
Name & address of editor : Dr. J. R. Rao
Division of Parasitology Indian Veterinary Research Institute,
Izatnagar-243 122 (UP)

32. LABORATORY ANIMALS INDIA*

Year of establishment : 1988
Published by : Laboratory Animal Science Association of India
Periodicity : Bi-annual
Name & address of editor : Dr. K. R. Bhardwaj
National Laboratory Animal Centre Central Drug Research Institute Lucknow-226001 (UP)

*** Out of Print**

33. INDIAN JOURNAL OF MEAT SCIENCE AND TECHNOLOGY*

Year of establishment : 1988
Published by : Indian Association of Meat Science & Technologies
Periodicity : Bi-annual
Name & address of editor : Dr. Nagendra Sharma
Division of Livestock Products Technology IVRI, Izatnagar-243 122 (UP)

***Out of Print**

34. THE JOURNAL OF BOMBAY VETERINARY COLLEGE

Year of establishment : 1989
Published by : College
Periodicity : Half-yearly
Name & address of editor : Dr. S. N. Naik
Bombay Veterinary College Parel, Mumbai (M.S.)

35. INDIAN JOURNAL OF VETERINARY ANATOMY

Year of establishment : 1989
Published by : Indian Association of Veterinary Anatomists

Periodicity : Bi-annual

Name & address of editor : Dr. Chandra Pal
Department of Anatomy College of Veterinary and Animal Sciences
Mathura-281 001

36. INDIAN JOURNAL OF COMPARATIVE MICROBIOLOGY, IMMUNOLOGY AND INFECTIOUS DISEASES

Year of establishment : 1988

Published by : Indian Association of Veterinary Mircobiologists, Immunologists & Specialists in Infectious Diseases

Periodicity : Bi-annual

Name & address of editor : Dr. K. C. Verma, Head
Division of Avian Diseases
Indian Veterinary Research Institute,
Izatnagar-243 122 (UP)

37. INDIAN JOURNAL OF ANIMAL PHYSIOLOGY

Year of establishment : 1992

Published by : Society of Animal Physiologists of India

Periodicity : Bi-annual

Name & address of editor : Dr. G.C. Georgie
Department of Animal Physiology
College of Veterinary Science
Hisar-125 004 (Haryana)

38. THE INDIAN JOURNAL OF VETERINARY RESEARCH

Year of establishment : 1992

Published by : Indian Association for the Advancement of Veterinary Research

Periodicity : Bi-annual

Name & address of editor	:	Dr. Rishendra Verma Senior Scientist Division of Bacteriology & Mycology Indian Veterinary Research Izatnagar-243 122 (UP)

39. INDIAN JOURNAL OF TOXICOLOGY

Year of establishment	:	1994
Published by	:	Camel Publishing House
Periodicity	:	Bi-annual
Name & address of editor	:	Dr. T.K. Gahlot Department of Surgery and Radiology College of Veterinary Science Bikaner-334001 (Raj)

40. THE INDIAN JOURNAl OF SMALL RUMINANTS

Year of establishment	:	1995
Published by	:	Indian Society for Sheep and Goat Production and Utilization
Periodicity	:	Bi-annual
Name & address of editor	:	Dr. S. Parthasarthy Senior Scientist Central Sheep & Wool Research Institute (Malpura, Distt: Tonk) AVIKANAGAR (via Jaipur) Rajasthan-304 501

TECHNICAL/POPULAR PERIODICALS

INDIAN FARMING

Year of establishment	:	1940
Published by	:	Indian Council of Agricultural Research (ICAR)
Periodicity	:	Monthly
Address	:	Editor Publication & Information Division Indian Council of Agricultural Research (ICAR) Krishi Anusandhan Bhavan, Pusa, New Delhi

INDIAN DAIRYMAN

Year of establishment	: 1948
Published by	: Indian Dairy Association
Periodicity	: Monthly
Address	: Ms Sheeba Chopra Indian Dairy Association IDA House, sector IV R. K. Puram, New Delhi-110002

GOSAMVARDHAN*

Year of establishment	: 1955
Published by	: Central Council of Gosamvardhan
Periodicity	: Monthly
Address	: 16 A Sandarshan Court Ajmeri Gate Extension, New Delhi

*Out of Print

CHEETAL

Year of establishment	: 1961
Published by	: The Wild Preservation Society of India
Periodicity	: Quarterly
Address	: Editor, Cheetal Wild Preservation Society 7, Astlay Hall Dehradun (UP)

INTENSIVE AGRICULTURE

Year of establishment	: 1964
Published by	: Ministry of Agriculture & Irrigation
Periodicity	: Monthly
Address	: Mr. Ravi Verma Directorate of Extension Ministry of Agriculture & Irrigation New Delhi-110001

POULTRY GUIDE

Year of establishment : 1964
Published by : Guide Group of Publications (India) Pvt. Ltd.
Periodicity : Monthly
Address : Mr. C. P. Narang
1700, Sector 4, Urban Estate
Gurgaon-122001 (Haryana)

ANIMAL CITIZEN

Year of establishment : 1965
Published by : Animal Welfare Board of India
Periodicity : Quarterly
Address : Editor
Animal Welfare Board of India 7, 2nd Cross Street, Venue Colony
Alwarpet, Chennai-600 018 (TN)

FARMER AND PARLIAMENT

Year of establishment : 1962
Published by : Farmers Parliamentary Forum
Periodicity : Monthly
Address : S. N. Bhalla
144, South Avenue
New Delhi

INDIAN FARMER'S DIGEST

Year of establishment : 1968
Published by : G. B. Pant University
Periodicity : Monthly
Address : Dr. S. G. Dwivedi
G. B. Pant University of Agriculture & Technology
Pantnagar-263 145 (UP)

POULTRY ADVISOR

Year of establishment : 1968
Published by : Private
Periodicity : Monthly
Address : Dr. S. Abdul Rahman
124/2, 7th "B" Main Road
Bangalore-560011

INDIAN POULTRY REVIEW

Year of establishment : 1978
Published by : Mr. G. N. Singh
Periodicity : Monthly
Address : Mr. G. N. Ghosh
57- B Townshed Road
Calcutta-700025

HARYANA FARMING

Year of establishment : 1971
Published by : CCS Haryana Agricultural University
Periodicity : Monthly
Address : Editor Directorate of Publications
Gandhi Bhawan,
CCS Haryana Agricultural University
Hisar-125 004

POULTRY TODAY

Year of establishment : 1972
Published by : Private
Periodicity : Monthly
Address : Amar Rudra
Ramkanai Adhikari Lane
Calcutta-700012 (W.B.)

LIVESTOCK ADVISOR

Year of establishment : 1975
Published by : T. A. Gaffar
Periodicity : Monthly
Address : Dr. R. S. Rafiuddin
97, St. John's Church Road
Bangalore-560 005

THE VETERINARIAN

Year of establishment : 1978
Published by : Private
Periodicity : Monthly
Address : Mrs Shireen Rahman
123, 7th B Main Road, IV Block
(West), Jaynagar, Bangalore-560011

FARMER'S JOURNAL*

Year of establishment : 1981
Periodicity : Monthly
Address : Yaspal Kapoor for Associated Journals Ltd, 2/1, E. N. S. Building, Rafi Marg
New Delhi-110001

POULTRY PUNCH

Year of establishment : 1984
Published by : Poultry Punch Publications (India) Pvt. Ltd.
Periodicity : Monthly
Address : Mr. B. S. Rana
25, Thyagraj Nagar Market
New Delhi-110003

RAKSHA TECHNICAL BULLETIN*

Year of establishment : 1985
Published by : Indian Immunologicals
Periodicity : Quarterly
Address : M/S Indian Immunologicals
11-4-657, Lakdi-ka-Pul
Hyderabad-4

***Out of Print**

ZOO'S PRINT

Year of establishment : 1986
Published by : Zoo Outreach Organisation
Periodicity : Monthly
Address : N. V. K. Ashraf
Zoo Outreach Organisation
PB 1683, 65, Bharathi Colony
Peelamedu
Coimbatore-641 004

POULTRY TODAY AND TOMORROW

Year of establishment : 1991
Published by : Private
Periodicity : Bi-annual
Address : Smt. Poonam Chaudhary
1314 HIG II (GF) Gaurav Nivas
Housing Board Colony
Sector 15 A, HISAR-125 001 (Haryana)

POULTRY FORTUNE

Year of establishment : 1992
Published by : Private
Periodicity : Monthly

Address : Mr. Z. A. Zazeer
8 A, 3rd Floor, Lenaine Estate
Abid Road, Gunfoundary
Hyderabad-500 001

PET INDIA

Year of establishment : 1985
Published by : Private, M/S Pet India
Periodicity : Monthly
Address : Dr. B. C. Ramakrishna
630, 17th "A" Main Road
6th Block, Koramangala
Bangalore-560 095

NATIONAL EGG COORDINATION COMMITTEE'S REVIEW

Year of establishment : 1996
Published by : National Egg Coordination Committee
Periodicity : Monthly
Address : Dr. G. S. Reddy
National Egg Coordination Committee
3-5-832, 3rd Floor, Baseerbagh
Hyderabad-500029 (A.P.)

POULTRY TIMES OF INDIA

Year of establishment : 1996
Published by : Private
Periodicity : Fortnightly
Address : Mr. Ravi Chawla
Hibiscus "A" 301-302 Plot 1189
Year Road, Next to Silvertcroft
Versova, Mumbai-400061 (M.S.)

LIVESTOCK INTERNATIONAL

Year of establishment : 1997
Published by : M/S Indian Herbs
Periodicity : Monthly
Address : Ms. Namitha Rao
C-503, UNESCO Assn Apts, 551p.
Extension, Delhi-110 092

INTAS POLIVET

Year of establishment : 1998
Published by : Intas Pharmaceuticals Ltd.
Periodicity : Bi-annual
Address : Dr. A. P. Mamtani
Chief Editor
Intas Pharmaceuticals Ltd.
A-74, Radha Krishna Park
Near Akota Stadium
Akota
VADODARA-390 020 (Gujarat)

NEWS PAPERS

PASHUDHAN

Year of establishment : 1980
Published by : Guide Group of Publications
Periodicity : Weekly
Address : Mr. C. P. Narang
20, Thyagrajnagar Market
(Lodi Road), NEW DELHI

PASHU JAGAT

Year of establishment : 1982
Published by : Bhartiya Boote Bhavan

Periodicity : Monthly
Address : Mr. S. K. Agrawal
21, Mangal Nagar
Saharanpur-247 001 (UP)

POULTRY FLAME

Year of establishment : 1982
Published by : Poultry Punch Publications (India) Pvt. Ltd.
Address : Mr. B. S. Rana
25, Thaygraj Nagar Market
New Delhi-110003

HINDI PERIODICALS

पशुप्रोषण

स्थापना : 1991
अवधि : त्रैमासिक
संपादक एवं पता : आर. बी. चौधरी
4/227 विकास नगर,
लखनऊ—226012

खेती

स्थापना : भारतीय कृषि अनुसंधान संस्थान
अवधि : मासिक
संपादक एवं पता : श्री कुलदीप शर्मा
प्रकाशन एवं सूचना विभाग
भारतीय कृषि अनुसंधान परिषद
पूसा, नई दिल्ली

वैटरनरी टूडे

स्थापना : 1992
अवधि : त्रैमासिक
संपादक एवं पता : नीरज कुमार वर्मा
1/10 आर. वी. सी. कांके राची,
विहार-834007

शालीहोत्र

अविधि	:	द्विमासिक
संपादक एवं पता	:	STO रमेश चन्द्र उपाध्याय शाली होत्र प्रकाशन मण्डलेश्वर जिला खरगौन—451221 (म. प्र.)

पोल्ट्री गाइड

अवधि	:	मासिक
संपादक एवं पता	:	सी. पी. नारंग 24, धागराज नगर मार्केट, नई दिल्ली

गौसम्र्बधन ●

स्थापना	:	1955
अवधि	:	मासिक
संपादक एवं पता	:	16 ए सैन्डीसन कोर्ट अजमेरी गेट एक्सटेंशन नई दिल्ली

● अब नही छपती ।

पशुधन अनुसंधान ●

स्थापना	:	1990
अवधि	:	छमाही
संपादकीय पता	:	राजबाषा अनुभाग भारतीय पशुचिकित्सा अनुसंधान संस्थान इज्जत नगर—243122 (उ. प्र.)

● अभी प्रकाशन स्थगित है।

Chapter - 13

ACADEMY, ICAR AND SOCIETY AWARDS

Sl.	Academy/Society	Name of Award
1.	Indian Council of Agricultural Research (ICAR)	1. Best Institution Award 2. Rafi Ahmed Kidwai Award for Agricultural Research 3. Fakhruddin Ali Ahmed Award for outstanding research in Tribal Areas 4. Vasant Rao Naik Award for Research Application in Agriculture 5. Jawaharlal Nehru Award for Post-graduate Agricultural Research 6. Outstanding Women Agricultural Scientist Award 7. Best KVK Awards for the Outstanding Extension Scientist 8. National Awards for out-standing teachers
2.	Indian Science Academy	FASc
3.	Indian National Science Academy	FNA
4.	National Academy of Sciences	FNASc
5.	National Academy of Agricultural Sciences	FNAASc
6.	National Academy of Veterinary Science	FNAVSc

Contd....

Sl.	Academy/Society	Name of Award
7.	Indian Veterinary Association [Awards for Best Paper published The Indian Vet. J.]	1. Dr. Siddique Award for Best Paper in Vety. Public Health 2. Late Dr. Rao Sahib Dr.V. R. Gopalakrishna Award for Best Paper in Animal Nutrition 3. Dr. T. Prabhakaran Award for Best Paper in Livestock Production Management 4. Smt Leelavathi Krishnarao Award for Best Paper in Small Ruminants 5. Dr. P. R. Krishna Iyer Award for Best Paper in Bacteriology 6. Alarsin Award for Best Paper in Medicine/Therapeutics/ Pharamacology 7. Dr. R. Eswaran Award 8. Dr. P. Krishnamurthi Medal for Best Short Communication 9. Shri Anjan K. Orugauti Medal for Best Paper in Physiology 10. Dr. P. R. Nilakantan Award 11. Dr. Rao Bahadur R. Swaminathan Iyer Award for Best Clinical Paper 12. Bishnu Sudama Award 13. Dr. K. S. Memorial Award for Best Research Paper in Bacteriology/ Virology/ Pathology 14. Dr. Ghanti A. Sastry Award Best Research Paper in Pathology 15. Prof. Nils Lagerlof Memorial Prize for Best Paper in Animal Reproduction.
8.	Indian Society for the Study of Reproduction	1. Prof. Nils Lagerlof Award & 2. G. B. Singh Award Best Paper 3. ISSAR Fellowship 4. Prof. C. R. Sane Oration Lecture 5. Dr. S. N. Luktuke Award for Best Presentation 6. Best Field Veterinarian
9.	Indian Association of - Comprataive Microbiology, Immunology & Specialists in Infectious Diseases	1. Dr. C. M. Singh Award for Best paper in Veterinary Microbiology

Contd....

Sl.	Academy/Society	Name of Award
		2. Dr. P. K. Uppal Young Scientist Travel Grant
		3. Late Dr. P. G. Pandey Oration Lecture
10.	Indian Society of Veterinary Biotechnology & Immunology	1. Dr. Richard Massilamony Oration Lecture
		2. Young Scientist Award
11.	Indian Association of Veterinary Pathologists	1. M/S SKM Animal Feed & Food Pvt. Ltd. Award
		& 2. Narmada Hatcheries Award for Best Presentation
		3. Dr. Ram Raksha Kiran Shukla Award for MVSc Thesis
		4. Dr. C. M. Singh Award for Best Paper in Veterinary Pathology
		5. Best poster presentation
		6. Vee Care Award for outstanding contribution of individual/institution during last three years
		7. Ventribiological Endowment Lecture on Diseases of Poultry.
12.	Indian Society of Veterinary Medicine	1. Late Sh. Ram Lal Agrawal Gold Medal for best work in Vety. Medicine/indigenous Vety. Medicine
		2. Young Scientist Award for Best Presentation
		3. Dr. P. L. Narayana Rao Gold Medal for Best contribution in research/ teaching
		4. Dr. D. C. Blood Gold Medal for teaching, research and other activities
		5. Best Clinical Paper Award
		6. ISVM Appreciation Award
		7. Smt. P.Z. Sharma Gold Medal for Canine Medicine
		8. Sri Matunga Jain Gowrak- sath Mandali Gold Medal for Bovine Medicine
		9. S. K. M. Gold Medal for Poultry Medicine
13.	Society of Toxicology, India	1. Fellowship STOX

Contd....

Sl.	Academy/Society	Name of Award
14.	Indian Association for the Advancement of Veterinary Research	1. Major (Mrs) Malika Trivedi IAAVR Award Research
		2. Prof. Ramraksha Kiran Shukla Award in Animal Health & Production
		3. Best Paper Award
		4. Fellow IAAVR
		5. Young Scientist IAAVR Award
		6. Late G. V. Narayankhedkar Memorial Award In Animal Husbandry
		7. Late Shyama Singh & Balamati Devi Memorial Award for excellence in Animal Health Care and Cover
		8. Shri Ahiylaya Mata Jeev Daya Mandal Trust Award for research on indigenous cows
15.	Indian Association for the Advancement of Veterinary Parasitology	1. Dr. J. P. Dubey Young Scientist Award for Research work.
16.	Indian Poultry Science Association	1. Kerala Chapter IPSA Award in Poultry Nutrition
		2. Prof. P. K. Pani Research Award in Poultry Genetics & Breeding & another in Immunology & Poultry Disease Resistance
		3. Dr. R. K. Shukla Young Scientist Award
		4. IPSA Fellowship

Chapter - 14

VETERINARY BIOLOGICAL INSTITUIONS

In India, the production of veterinary biologicals at Indian Veterinary Research Institutes dates back to 1898. The institute produced and released a number of antisera against rinderpest, haemorrhagic septicaemia, anthrax, tetanus and black quarter and mallen at Mukteshwar (Kumaon) during 1898-1910. Later, large scale production of biological was undertaken by the Imperial Veterinary Serum Institute, Izatnagar. In order to cope up with the increasing demand of veterinary biologicals, various States have instituted biological production units.

1. DIVISION OF BIOLOGICAL PRODUCTS IVRI, Izatnagar-243 122 (UP)

The Division of Biological Products came into existence as Imperial Serum Institute in 1930. In 1936, with the re-organisation of the institute, the division was renamed as the Division of Biological Products. In 1950's the Division was strengthened with the help of WHO and infrastructural facilities was created by remodelling of building and through addition of laboratories.

Bacterial Vaccines

Live Vaccine

(1) Anthrax spore vaccine

(2) *Brucella abortus* strain 19 living vaccine

Killed/Inactivated Vaccines

(1) Black Quarter Vaccine
(2) Haemorrhagic septicaemia vaccine
(3) *Salmonella abortus equi* vaccine
(4) Enterotoxaemia vaccine
(5) Multicomponent Clostridial vaccine

Viral Vaccines
Live Vaccine

(1) Tissue culture rinderpest vaccine
(2) Sheep-pox cell-culture vaccine
(3) Rabies vaccine, Flury strain LEP
(4) Horsesickness vaccine
(5) Swine-fever-lapinised vaccine
(6) Ranikhet disease F strain vaccine
(7) Ranikhet disease R_2B vaccine
(8) Fowl pox vaccine, chicken embryo virus
(9) Marek's disease vaccine
(10) Avian Influenza bronchitis vaccine

Killed/inactivated vaccines

(1) Foot and Mouth Disease vaccine
(2) Rabies vaccine (inactivated) 5% BPL
(3) Rabies vaccine (inactivated) cell-culture
(4) Canine distemper vaccine
(5) Infectious bursal disease vaccine (inactivated)

Antigens

(1) PPD tuberculin
(2) Avian tuberculin
(3) *Brucella abortus* coloured antigen
(4) *Brucella abortus* plain antigen

(5) ABR antigen
(6) Mallein PPD
(7) Johnin
(8) *Salmoenlla pullorum* coloured antigen
(9) *Salmonella pullorum* plain antigen
(10) *Salmonella abortus equi* 'H' antigen

IVRI REGIONAL STATION, HEBBAL, BANGALORE

(1) Foot and Mouth Disease Vaccine

2. INSTITUTE OF ANIMAL HEALTH AND VETERINARY BIOLOGICAL PRODUCTS

Hebbal, Bangalore-560024
Tel: 3331502, 2332442; Gram:ANIHEALTH
Year of establishment : 1926

Bacterial vaccines
Live vaccine

(1) *Brucella abortus* strain-19 vaccine

Killed/inactivated vaccine

(1) Haemorrhagic septicaemia vaccine
(2) Black Quarter vaccine
(3) Enterotoxaemia vaccine
(4) Anthrax vaccine
(5) Duck *Pasteurella* vaccine

Viral vaccine
Live vaccine

(1) Rinderpest tissue culture vaccine
(2) Sheep pox tissue culture vaccine
(3) R_2B vaccine
(4) Ranikhet 'F' vaccine
(4) Fowl pox vaccine
(5) Pigeon pox vaccine

Killed/inactivated vaccine

(1) Antirabies vaccine (Pre)
(2) Antirabies vaccine (Post)

Antigens

(1) *Salmonella pullorum* coloured antigen
(2) *Brucella abortus* rose Bengal plate test antigen
(3) *Brucella* plain antigen (True test antigen)
(4) *Brucella abortus* plain antigen (Marcaptoethanol test)
(5) *Brucella abortus* milk ring antigen (Haemotoxylin stained)
(6) *Brucella abortus* milk ring antigen (Tetrazolium stained)

Diluents

(1) TCRPV diluent
(2) Poultry vaccine diluent
(3) Pox diluent

3. VETERINARY BIOLOGICAL AND RESEARCH INSTITUTE
Shantinagar, Hyderabad-500028 (A.P.)
Phone: 3316366; Gram: BIOVET
Year of establishment : 1944

Bacterial vaccines
Live vaccine
(1) Anthrax spore vaccine

Killled/inactivated vaccine

(1) Haemorrhagic speticaemia (Alum precipitated and oil adjuvant)
(2) Black Quarter vaccine
(3) Enterotoxaemia vaccine

Viral vaccine
Live vaccine

(1) Rinderpest tissue culture vaccine
(2) Sheep pox vaccine

(3) Ranikhet disease "K" vaccine
Ranikhet disease "F" vaccine

(4) Fowl pox vaccine

Killed/inactivated vaccine

(1) Antirabies vaccine (Prophylactic & Postbite)

4. INSTITUTE OF VETERINARY PREVENTIVE MEDICINE
Ranipet (Tamil Nadu)-632402

Year of establishment : 1932

Bacterial vaccines

Live vaccines

(1) Anthrax spore vaccine

(2) *Brucella abortus* strain 19 vaccine

Killed/inactivated vaccine

(1) Haemorrhagic speticaemia vaccine alum treated

(2) Haemorrhagic septicaemia oil adjuvant vaccine

(3) Black Quarter

(4) Bovine lymphangitis vaccine

(5) Enterotoxaemia Vaccine

Viral vaccine

(1) Rinderpest goat adapted tissue vaccine

(2) Tissue culture rinderpest vaccine

(3) Sheep pox vaccine

(4) Rabies Flury strain LEP vaccine

(5) Ranikhet disease vaccine- Kamrov strain

(6) Ranikhet disease vaccine F & Labota strain

(7) Fowl pox vaccine, pigeon pox virus

Killed/inactivated vaccine

(1) Canine distemper vaccine

(2) Fowl pox vaccine

Antigens

1. California mastitis (CMT) test
2. *Brucella abortus* coloured antigen
3. *Brucella abortus* plain antigen
4. ABR antigen
5. *Brucella melitensis* tube antigen
6. *Salmonella pullorum* coloured antigen
7. PPLO antigen

5. INSTITUTE OF VETERINARY BIOLOGICAL PRODUCTS
Ganeshkhind Road, Aundh, Pune (M.S.)

Tel: 375632; Fax: 357962

Year of establishment: 1947

Bacterial vaccines

Live vaccine

(1) Anthrax spore vaccine
(2) *Brucella* strain -19 vaccine

Killed/inactivated vaccines

(1) Black Quarter vaccine
(2) Haemorrhagic septicaemia oil adjuvant vaccine
(3) Haemorrhagic septicaemia alum treated
(4) Botulinum vaccine
(5) Enterotoaxemia vaccine
(6) Spirochaetosis vaccine

Viral vaccine
Live vaccine

(1) Ranikhet disease (Mukteshwar)
(2) Ranikhet disease (Lasota strain)
(3) Fowl pox
(4) Sheep pox

(5) Anti rabies vaccine (5%) ML
(6) Anti rabies vaccine (20%) ML
(7) Tissue culture rinderpest vaccine
(8) TCRP
(9) Marek's disease

Antigen

1. *Brucella* RBPT antigen
2. *Brucella* plain antigen
3. *Salmonella* coloured antigen
4. California mastitis test reagent

6. HARAYAN VETERINARY VACCINE INSTITUTE
Hisar-125 004 (Haryana)

Tel:37093; Gram: VACCINE
Year of establishment : 1948

Bacterial vaccines
Killed/inactivated vaccine

(1) HS alum vaccine
(2) HS oil adjuvanted vaccine
(3) Enterotoaxemia vaccine
(4) Black Quarter vaccine

Viral vaccines
Live vaccine

(1) Sheep pox vaccine
(2) Lap. swine fever vaccine
(3) F1 Ranikhet disease vaccine
(4) R_2B Ranikhet disease vaccine
(5) Fowl pox vaccine

Killed/inactivated vaccine

(1) Antirabic 5% vaccine
(2) Antirabic 20% vaccine (Prophylatic single dose)

7. INSTITUTE OF ANIMAL HEALTH & VETERINARY BIOLOGICALS

Rasalpur, Mhow (M.P.)-453 446

Year of establishment : 1949

Bacterial vaccines
Live vaccine

(1) Anthrax spore vaccine

Killed/inactivated vaccines

(1) HS alum precipitated vaccine
(2) Black Quarter vaccine
(3) HS oil adjuvant vaccine
(4) Enterotoxaemia vaccine
(5) Spirochaetosis

Viral vaccines
Live vaccine

(1) Ranikhet regular
(2) Ranikhet disease "F" strain
(3) Fowl pox
(4) Sheep pox (TC)
(5) Marek's disease
(6) Swine-fever

Killed/inactivated vaccines

(1) Antirabies vaccine (SD)
(2) Antirabies (MD)
(3) Tissue culture Rinderpest vaccine

8. INSTITUTE OF ANIMAL HEALTH & PRODUCTION

Patna-14, Bihar

Year of establishemnt : 1953

Bacterial vaccines
Live vaccine

(1) Anthrax spore vaccine (live)

Killed/inactivated vaccines

(1) Haemorrhagic septicaemia alum treated vaccine
(2) Black Quarter vaccine

Viral vaccine
Live vaccine

(1) Ranikhet disease vaccine R_2 B strain (live)
(2) Ranikhet disease vaccine, F1 strain (live)
(3) Fowl pox vaccine, pigeon pox virus

9. PUNJAB VETERINARY VACCINE INSTITUTE
Punjab Agricultural University, Ludhiana
Tel : 401439; Gram : Vcacines

Year of establishment : 1973

Bacterial vaccines

(1) HS alum-precipitated vaccine
(2) HS oil adjuvant vaccine
(3) Black Quarter vaccine
(4) Enterotoxaemia vaccine

Viral vaccines
Live vaccine

(1) Ranikhet R_2B vaccine
(2) Ranikhet F strain
(3) Fowl pox
(4) Swine fever

Killed/inactivated vaccines

(5) Antirabic vaccine 5% (BPL)
(6) Antirabic vaccine 2%

Antigen

Salmonella pullorum **coloured antigen**

10. ANIMAL VACCINE INSTITUTE

Near Water Tank, Sector 28, Gandhinagar-382028 (Gujarat)

Year of estbalishment : 1976

Bacterial vaccines

(1) Haemorrhagic septicaemia alum precipitated

(2) Black Quarter

(3) Enterotoxaemia

Viral vaccines

(1) Ranikhet disease "F" strain

(2) Ranikhet disease R_2B strain

(3) Fowl pox vaccine

(4) Sheep pox vaccine

Antigens

(1) *Salmonella pullorum* coloured antigen

(2) *Brucella* plain as well as coloured antigen under experimental batch

11. INSTITUTE OF ANIMAL HEALTH AND BIOLOGICAL PRDOUCTS

Zakura, Srinagar; Tel (O)455091

Year of establishment : 1982

Bacterial vaccines

Live vaccine

(1) Anthrax

(2) Black Quarter

(3) Haemorrahgic septicaemia

(4) FDC

Viral vaccine
Live vaccine

Ranikhet disease

12. MIRDULA SARABHAI INSTITUTE OF ANIMAL HEALTH AND BIOLOGICAL PRODUCTS

R. S. Pura (Jammu) J &K State Tel:50217

Year of establishment : 1989

Bacterial vaccines

(1) HS vaccine

(2) Black Quarter vaccine

Viral vaccine

(1) Antirabic vaccine (Prophylactic & Post-bite)

(2) Ranikhet disease vaccine [F strain, LaSota, R_2 B strain]

(3) Fowl pox

(4) Autogenous liver homogenised vaccine for control of hydropericardiu/IBM in poultry

13. ORISSA BIOLOGICAL PRODUCTS INSTITUTE

Berhampur-760001 Dist : Ganjam (Orissa)

Year of establishment : 1982

Bacterial vaccines

(1) HS alum adjuvant vaccine

(2) Black quarter vaccine

Viral vaccines : Nil

Antigens : Nil

14. INSTITUTE OF VETERINARY BIOLOGICALS

Guwahati (Assam)-781022

Year of establishment : 1949-50

Bacterial vaccines

Live vaccine

(1) Anthrax spore vaccine

Killed/inactivated vaccines

(1) Black Quarter vaccine

(2) Haemorrhagic septicaemia vaccine

(3) Enterotoxaemia vaccine

Viral vaccines
Live vaccine

(1) Rinderpest goat adapted tissue culture vaccine
(2) Swine fever lapinised vaccine
(3) Ranikhet F strain vaccine
(4) Ranikhet R_2B vaccine

Killed/inactivated vaccines

(1) Rabies vaccine (inactivated 5%)
(2) Rabies vaccine (inactivated 20%)
(3) Fowl pox vaccine
(4) Fowl pox vaccine, pigeon pox virus
(5) Duck plague vaccine

15. BIOLOGICAL PRODUCTS SECTION
37, Belgachia, Calcutta (West Bengal)

Year of establishment : 1985

Bacterial vaccines

Live vaccine

(1) Anthrax spore vaccine

Killed/inactivated vaccine

(2) Haemorrahgic septicaemia vaccine
(2) Fowl cholera vaccine

Viral vaccines
Live vaccine

(1) Rinderpest goat adapted tissue vaccine
(2) Rabies Flury strain LEP
(3) Swine fever lapinised
(4) Ranikhet disease F strain
(5) Ranikhet R_2 strain

Killed/inactivated vaccine

(1) Haemorrhgaic septicaemia vaccine
(2) Fowl cholera vaccine

Viral vaccines

(1) Rinderpest goat adapted tissue vaccine
(2) Rabies Flury strain LEP
(3) Swine fever lapinised
(4) Ranikhet disease F strain
(5) Ranikhet R_2B strain

Killed/inactivated vaccine

(1) Rabies vaccine (20%, inactivated)
(2) Fowl pox vaccine
(3) Fowl pox vaccine, pigeon pox vaccine
(4) Duck plague vaccine

16. REGIONAL VETERINARY BIOLOGICAL INSTITUTE, JAIPUR (RAJASTHAN)

Year of establishment : 1957

Bacterial vaccines

Live vaccine

(1) Anthrax spore vaccine

Killed/inactivated vaccine

(1) Black Quarter vaccine
(2) Haemorrhagic septicaemia vaccine
(3) Enterotoxaemia vaccine
(4) Spirochaetosis vaccine

Viral vaccines
Live vaccines

(1) Rinderpest goat adapted tissue vaccine
(2) Ranikhet disease R_2B strain vaccine
(3) Ranikhet disease F strain vaccine

17. VETERINARY BIOLOGICAL INSTITUTE, Palode (Kerala)

Year of establishment :

Bacterial vaccines

(1) Haemorrhagic septicaemia alum treated vaccine

(2) Black Quarter vaccine

Viral vaccine

Live vaccine

(1) Ranikhet Disease F strain vaccine

(2) Ranikhet disease R_2B strain vaccine

Killed/inactivated

(1) Fowl-pox vaccine

Chapter - 15

VETERINARIANS AND VETERINARY SERVICE

The esrtwhile USSR had the largest number of veterinarians in the world i.e., 80,000 while USA is the second largest country in the world having the strength of 36,000 vets (FAO, 1979). India ranks third having 20,000 vets. Brazil, Germany and UK follows in that order. It is postulated while calculating the need of veterinarians, two factors viz; human (H) and Livestock (LA) should be considered since the ultimate objective of veterinary service is to serve the human through livestock development. Table 1 describes the projected need of veterinarians by 1990 (FAO, 1990).

Table 1 : Projected need of veterinarians by 1990, India

	1980	*GR*		*1990* *GR*	
1. Govt. Veterinarians	14,000	3%	18,200	5%	21,000
2. Centre/State Administrative Veterinarians	1,500	3%	1,950	5%	2,250
3. Teaching/Research Veterinarians	1,400	5%	2,100	15%	3,500
4. Industry Veterinarians (Feed, Drug, Biologicals, Poultry)	1,350	10%	2,700	20%	4,050
5. Cooperatives/Boards/ Pvt. Bodies (NDDB,BAIF etc.)	1,100	5%	1,650	7%	1,870
6. Bank/Insurance Veterinarians	250	10%	500	20%	750
7. Military Veterinarians	300	3%	390	3%	390
8. Meat Inspection Veterinarians or Meat Inspectors	150	6%	240	10%	300

Contd....

9.	Private Practitioners (Large, small animals, equines)	100	15%	250	20%	300
10.	Laboratory Animal Vets	50	10%	100	15%	125
11.	Retired Veterinarians	600	3%	850	3%	1025
12.	Others (200 wildlife, Pub. Health)	50	4%	70	4%	70
	Total Vets:	20,850		29,000		35,640
	Growth 10 Y		39%		70%	
	Annual growth		4%		7%	
	Human Population		684 m			820 m

As per the FAO/OIE (1996) the present position of Veterinarians in India is as follows:

Government Officials (Central, local)	=	29500
In labs, universities, training institutions	=	2830
Private Practitioners	=	1055
Other Veterinarians	=	1025
Total		34410

Singh (1998) published an overview of animal health services in India (Proc. Seminar on Poverty Alleviation through Livestock and Development, 3 May 1997, Delhi Veterinary Association, New Delhi). During the last two decades there has been a significant increase in the number of veterinary professionals (Table 2).

Table 2 : Availability of manpower for animal health services

	1981	*1985*	*1990*	*1993*	*%change in 1993 over 85*
No. of Professional Veterinarians	18000	25300	29900	33600	32.81
(a) Govt. Jobs	-	90.90	86.62	86.01	25.65
(b) Private	-	1.19	1.92	2.68	200.00
(c) Labs	-	5.93	8.53	8.33	86.67
(d) Others	-	1.98	2.93	2.98	200.00
VLUs per veterinarian	15428	12189	10515	9359	-
No. of veterinary auxiliaries	40000	51000	61500	65400	28.24
VLU per auxiliary	6862	6047	5112	4808	-
Ratio of Govt. to private practitioners	-	76.67	45.04	32.11	

Source : Singh (1998), VLU = Veterinary Livestock Unit

As it was thought in old days that a Veterinarian's prime aim is to treat horses, hence, they were called 'horse doctors'. With the lopsided growth and progress of the profession in India, the veterinarians tasks have increased manifold over the centuries. Probably, the veterinary profession has been well appreciated by the society and a veterinarian is required to serve the divergent areas viz; pharmaceuticals, rural banks, insurance companies, paramedical departments, laboratory animal houses, government departments besides universities, colleges, and institutes. The potential of veterinary services has increased due to the ramifications of the subject specilization. In India, veterinary services are yet to be raised to a high profile. Veterinary profession is entering the 21st Century and as such veterinarians have to address challenging tasks and have to compete globally, particularly in rendering health services. They have to face new technologies and information explosion, of which they will make best use. In India, there is a need to assess the public visibility about veterinarians. The ethics are to be adhered to by the veterinarians. Veterinarian of today is much more exposed to superspecialization. His services can no longer be undermined and ignored by the society.

Singh, Rajendra, Birthal, P.S. and Rathore, B.S. (1998) Review of animal health services in India. Indian J. Anim. Sci. 68 : 420-424.

Chapter - 16

COUNTRY'S LIVESTOCK AND POULTRY

India is endowed with the immense wealth of livestock and poultry with so much diverse breeds. Therefore, livestock and poultry constitute a rich and vital resource for the country which may help in alleviation of poverty and may provide ample employment. Some of the very important facts about this sectors are as follows:

* The average land holding of small and marginal farmers involved in animal husbandry is between 1/2 acre to 2 acres.
* The gross value of output from the livestock sector was Rs. 797 million during 1994-95 or 26% of the value of the output of the Agriculture sector.
* The production of milk for 1995-96 and 1996-97 has been set at 66.2 million tonnes and 69 million tonnes respectively.
* The export of buffalo meat went up from 8.25 lakh tonnes in 1992-93 to 11.61 lakh tonnes.
* The production of 27,000 million eggs and 300 million broilers during 1994 was an all time high.
* The annual requirement of feed and fodder is estimated to be 25.4 million tonnes of concentrates, 353 million tonnes of green fodder (Source: Pashudhan, Vol. 12, Aug 1997,p.6).

The data on livestock population is provided by the Quinquennial Livestock Census through numerical enumeration with break up according to sex, breed, age etc. The first Census of cattle was conducted in British India in the year 1919-20. Livestock population in the country has increased by 0.1% from 4196 lakhs in 1982 Census to 4453 lakhs in the 1987 Census. During the period the cattle population in the country has increased by 3.7% from 1925 lakhs to 1977 lakhs and buffalo population has increased by 8.9% from 698 lakhs to 700 lakhs.

Livestock Census (1992) [In Millions]

[Source:Livestock Census, Directorate of Economics and Statistics, 1992, Deptt. of Animal Husbandry & Dairying, Ministry of Agriculture, Govt. of India, New Delhi].

1.	Cattle	204.53	2.	Buffaloes	83.50
3.	Sheep	50.80	4.	Goats	115.28
5.	Horse & Ponies	0.82	6.	Mules	0.20
7.	Donkey	0.97	8.	Camel	1.03
9.	Pigs	12.79	10.	Others (Yaks Mithun 126	0.06
11.	Poultry	307.07	12.	Dogs	21.77

Tables 1 and 2 describe a comparison of livestock population versus world and availability per capita of various animals products.

Table1 : Livestock population in India and world-1995 (In million)

Species	*World*	*India*		*Rank*
Cattle	1295.47	193	(14.9%)	1
Buffalo	150.14	78.83	(52.5%)	1
Sheep	1081.29	44.81	(4.14%)	5
Goat	627.01	118.3	(18.87%)	1
Pig	897.1	11.78	(1.31%)	—
Poultry	12273	435	(3.54%)	—

Source : FAO Quarterly Bull. of Staistics, 1995;

Figures in parentheses indicate percentage to world population.

Table 2 : Availability and deficit of livestock products in India

Com-modity	Per capita 1994	availability 2000 AD	ICMR Recomm-endation	Expected per capita deficit in 2000AD
Milk	193 g/day	240 g/day	250 g/day	10 g/day
Egg	30 eggs/ annum	41 eggs/annum	180 eggs/annum	139 eggs/annum
Meat	1.45 kg/annum	2.26 kg/annum	10.95 kg/annum	8.69 kg/annum

Source :Patel (1993) and Ranjhan (1995) Adopted from V. Ramakumar[1997] Seminar on Poverty alleviation through Livestock Development, New Delhi.

The livestock and poultry should come up as an industry in India and there is yet to a lot for the upliftment of productivity of animals.

Chapter - 17

VETERINARY LIBRARIES

NATIONAL LIBRARY OF VETERINARY SCIENCE

There is a National Library of Veterinary Science located at Indian Veterinary Research Institute, Izatnagar. This library has the largest collection of veterinary literature of both past and present in the form of journals both Indian and foreign, post-graduate thesis, foreign journals and rare publications. The library has got an Archives Section and Hindi Section. Library has also got latest hardware and software packages to handle library related activities. Facilities of CD-ROM net with various CD drives is also available. Establishment of V-set is in process to have collaboration with other research institutions. Introduction of multimedia PC's with sound blaster card, speaker, head phones and audiovisual CD-ROM aids for voice recording system for lecture demonstration are some facilities which are shortly to be created. Facilities of reprography is also available.

INSTITUTE AND UNIVERSITY LIBRARIES

Each State Agricultural University or Institute has got one library which also includes section for veterinary and animal science books, journals and other periodicals. Facilities of reprography are available in general.

COLLEGE LIBRARIES

Some of veterinary colleges do have a library which specifically provide books, journals, magazines etc. relating to veterinary science and animal husbandry.

DIVISIONAL LIBRARIES

Each division particularly at Indian Veterinary Research Institute at Izatnagar and its regional campus and stations has got a library which is specifically designed to meet the demand of specialized disciplines and acts as a readily available access to that subject.

ACCESS TO LIBRARIES

Access to libraries is not restricted. National Library of Veterinary Science or Central University Libraries or College Libraries have cataloguing system. Books, journals etc are shelved separately. These libraries also have a New Arrival Section which markedly displays newly procured editions of books. Some libraries have News Paper section. Modern facilities like reprography and computerized services are now available which make reader's job easy.

Chapter - 18

PUBLICATIONS

ICAR

The following publications may be obtained from Publication and Information Department, ICAR, Krishi Anusandhan Bhavan, Pusa, New Delhi.

Bhalerao, G. S. [1935] Helminth parasites of the domesticated animals in India. 365 p. Rs.7.75 (Sci. Monogr. 6).

Selected Clinical Articles (Pt.1) (14p, 50P) Misc. Bull. 8

1. Sharma, G. K. [1936] An interesting outbreak of variola vaccinia in milch cattle at Lahore
2. Kaura, R. L. [1936] An unusual case of navicular disease
3. Sharma, G. K. [1936] Super numerary teats in buffalo cows

Selected Clinical Articles (Pt.II) (19p, Rs.1.25) Misc. Bull. 15.

1. Sharma, G. K. [1936] Congenital corneal dermoid in a calf.
2. Kaura, R. L. and Iyer, S. G. [1936] Peculiar nervous derangement in a fowl infected with Ranikhet Disease Virus.
3. Sharma, G. K. and Khan, G.S. [1936] Atrophic cirrhosis of the liver and ascites in a ram
4. Mangrulkar, M. Y. [1936] Urinary calculus in the rabbit.

Selected Clinical Articles (Pt.III) (9p, 56P), Misc. Bull. 33

1. Rahim-Uddin, M. [1940] Few cases of Johne's disease in sheep.
2. Uttangi, C. D. [1940] A case of pregnancy in the mammary gland.
3. Nathani, R. C. and Sankaranarayanam, N. S. [1940] An unusual granuloma on the prepuce of a bull.

Agriculture & Animal Husbandry in India

1935-36; [1937] Rs.4.50

1936-37; [1939] Rs.7.00

1937-38; [1940] Rs.5.87

1938-39; [1941] Rs.6.00

Kartha, K. P. R. Comp. Milk records of cattle in approved dairy farms in India [1938]. 170p., Rs. 2.75 (Misc. Bull. 18).

Memorandum on the Development of Agriculture and Animal Husbandry in India [1944] Advisory Board of ICAR (79p. 56P)

Animal Disease Investigation [1947] (32p, Rs.1.50) (Misc. Bull. 65).

Brief survey of some of the important breeds of cattle in India.[1950] Pt.2 Prize winners at the First All India cattle show. Ed.2, Rs.1.37, 30 plates (Misc. Bull.24).

Definition of characteristics of Dhanni and Khillari cattle and Nili, Ravi and Surti buffaloes. [1950] Edn.2. 220, Rs.1.50 (Misc. Bull., 47).

Definition of characteristics of Kangayam, Khillari and Tharaparkar cattle and Nili and Surti buffaloes. Ed. 2 Rev. Delhi, Manager of Publications. 22p. rs.2.50.

Definition of characteristic of seven breeds of cattle of all India importance. Ed.3., 14p+xxvi plates, 75p (Bull.27).

Brief survey of some of the important breeds of cattle in India. [1951] Pt. 3 Prize winners at the 2nd and 3rd All India Cattle show. Ed.2, Rs. 2.00 (Misc. Bull. 46).

Dehorning of cattle [1952] 3p. 6p (Inf. Leaf.17).

Agriculture and Animal Husbandry Research.[1929-1946]. Part II. (1952), 190p. 50P.

Anand, D. M. [1953] Use balanced rations for cattle. 4p., 6P (Inf. Pamph. 37).

Sen, K. C. [1953] Animal Nutrition Research in India. Animal Husbandry Manual (370p, Rs.15.00 (Macmillian & Co.) for ICAR.

How to control Rinderpest. 2p 6P (Inf. Leafl. 38).

Mohan, R. N. [1954] Control of helminth parasites with special reference to livestock farms (49p, 50P (Rev. Ser.9).

Bakriyon ke lye rahane ka sthan (Hindi) 4p, 6P (Sooch Patra, 51).

Seetharaman, C. [1956] Ranikhet disease in poultry. 12p. 25P. (Res. ser. 9) Rev. 1960, 19p, 50P (Tech. Bull. AH, 3).

Kartha, K. P. R. [1957] Breeds of cattle in India. 52p, 50P (Misc. Bull. 32)

Mathur, A.C. [1957] Common ailments in cattle. 30p. 50P (Bull.23).

Bawa, H. S. [1957] Livestock products. 42p. 50P (Rev. Ser. 17).

Sen, K.C. [1957] Nutritive values of Indian cattle feeds and the feeding of animals. Ed.4, 46p. Rs. 1.25 (Misc. Bull. 25).

Kartha, K. P. R. [1958] Breeds of cattle in India. 52 p., 50P (Misc. Bull. 48).

Research in Animal Husbandry- A Review of work done during 1929-1954. [1962] 473p.

Lall, H.K. [1954] Goat keeping for profit. 32p. 25P (M. Bull, 4).

Housing goats [1954] 6P Inf. Pamph. 51).

Mohan, R. N. [1956] Animal Husbandry Education in India (40p. 25P (Central Scheme).

Lall, H.K. [1956] Bakripalan. 36p (Krishi Pustakmala Pushpa, 4).

Lall, H. K. [1956] Breeds of sheep in the Indian Union. 39p. Rs.2.87. (Misc. Bull. 75).

Bovine Stars of India [1957] All India Cattle show. (29p, Rs.2.37) Misc. Bull. 82.

Lall, H. K. [1957] Diagnosis of tuberculosis in animals with special reference to the tuberculin test. 22p. 30P (Rev. Ser.18). Revised in 1973.

Sen, K. C. and Ray, S. C. [1957] Principles of feeding farm animals. 27p. 37P (Rev. Ser. 15).

Khot, S. S. [1957] Sheep and Wool in India. 58p, 50P.

Khot, S. S. [1957] Better profits from sheep. 6p, 6P. (Inf. Leaflet, 80).

Iyer, S. G. [1958] Selecting Poultry Birds for Breeding. (6p, 6P(Inf. Leafl. 89)

Khot, S. S. [1958] Bhed palan se adhik labh (Hindi) 5p. 6P (Sooch Patra, 80).

Hoek, F. H. and Noorul, H. [1958] How to utilize carcasses. 36p. 50P. (M. Bull. 47).

Lall, J. M. [1958] Johne's Disease in cattle, sheep and goats. 27p. 55P. (Res. Ser. 19) Reprint, 1963, 25p, 70P.

Randhawa, M. S. [1958] Agriculture and Animal Husbandry in India (364p, Rs.15.00).

Dhanda, M. R. and Sharma, G. L. [1958] Incidence of anerobic infections in sheep. 21p. 75P (Rev. Ser., 26).

Dhanda, M. R. and Sharma, G. L. [1958] Investigation of mastitis in India. 41p. Rs.1.00 (Res. Ser. 35).

Kaura, R. L. [1958] Swine husbandry and piggery products. 53p. Rs.1.30. (Rev. Ser. 27).

Sen, S. K. [1959] Chemotherapy of animal trypanosomiasis (a resume of literature) 210p, Rs.9.50 (Sci. Mong. 22).

Bhatia, H. N. [1960] Coordination of Animal Husbandry Research in India. Vol.1 Pt.1 Animal Breeding, (1960) 41p., Vol.1 Pt.II-Animal Diseaees and Pests (1960), 106 p. Vol.1, Pt.III-Animal Nutrition, (1960), 70p.

Vol.I Pt.IV-Dairy Science (1960), 38 p.

Vol.I Pt.VI-Poultry Science, 1961, 35 p.

Srivastava, J.S. and Khera, R. C. [1960] Text Book of Animal Husbandry [1960] 198p.

Definitions of characteristics of cattle and buffalo breeds in India [1960]. 67p.+xvi Rs.3.00 (Misc. Bull. 86).

Agrawal, A. C. [1961] Production of wholesale meat in India. 84p, 60P.

Sen, S. K. and Fletcher, T. B. [1962] Veterinary entomology and acarology for India. 668p, 232 fig. 50 plates Rs.20.00.

Randhawa, M. S. [1962] Agriculture & Animal Husbandry in India. Rev Ed. 1962, xiii, 342p.

Chaudhari, R. P. [1962] Insect parasites of livestock and their control. 43p. Rs.1.30 (Res. ser., 29).

Randhawa, M.S. [1963] Bharat Mein Krishi Aur Pashupalan (Hindi) Translated by O.P. Sharma (368p, Rs.11.75).

Chaudhari, R. P. [1963] Pashuon ke parjiviki keet-Rog aur unki roktham (Hindi). 64p Rs.1.00 (Pustak, 12).

Nanda, P.N. [1963] Camels and their management. 17p, 75p (Rev. Ser.16).

Sen, K.C. and Anantha Krishnan, C. P. [1963] Dairy ke pashuon ka ahar aur unka dugdhkal (Hindi). 36p. 85P (Pustak Pushpa, 11).

Seetharaman, C. and Singh, K. C.[1963] Veterinary Biological Products and Their Use. 117p, Rs. 7.50.

Amble, V. N., Khandekar, N. C. and Garg, J. N. [1964] Statistical studies on breeding data of Beetal goats. (70p, Rs.4.00 (Res. ser.,38).

Deo, P. G. [1964] Roundworms of poultry. 146p. Rs.7.75 (Anim. Husb. ser.3.).

Anatomy of the ox with comparative notes on the horse, dog and fowl.[1964] 760p. Rs.50.

Kaura, R. L. [1965] Gosadans in India. 35p. 352

Sen, K.C. Nutritive values of Indian cattle feeds and the feeding of animals. (Revised by S.N. Ray, 1964. 133p. Rs.6.30) (Bill.25) Ed. 6 (Repr), 1971, 133p. Rs.6.30. Revised by S. N. Ray and S. K. Ranjhan [1978] 92p.

Singh Gajjan [1965] Artificial Insemination of Cattle in India. (44p, Rs.1.60) Tech. Bull. (A.H.), 1.

Bawa, H. S. and Bhote, R. A. [1966] Livestock products production and utilization. Revised ed. 49p, Rs.2.30. (Tech. Bull (AH),5).

Gangulee, P.C., Sharma, G. L. and Sen, G.P. [1967] Problem of Brucellosis in India. 220p, Rs.1.30 (Tech. Bull (AH), 7).

Khera, S.S. and Sharma, G. L. [1967] Important exotic diseases of livestock including poultry. viii+185p.

Kaura, R. L. and Bhatia, H. M. [1968] Contagious and parasitic diseases of sheep. 44p.

Sharma, G. L., Ranjit Sen and Mathur, T. N. [1968] Diagnostic techniques in Brucellosis. 10p (Tech. Bull. (AH), 9).

Sen, K. C. and Ananthakrishnan, C. P. [1968] Nutrition and lactation in dairy cattle. 49p, Rs.1.50 (Tech. Bull. (AH), 10).

Seetharaman, C. [1969] Murgiyon ka Ranikhet rog (Hindi) 23p. 90P.

Singh, D.,Rajagopalan, M. and Maini, J.S. [1970] Monograph on estimation of wool production. 43p. Rs.2.60.

Singh, D., Murthy, V. V. R. and Goel, B.B.P.S. [1970] Monograph on estimation of milk production. 80p. Rs.4.10.

Dhanda, M.R. and Sen, G.P. [1972] Haemorrhagic septicaemia and allied conditions in sheep, goats, pigs and poultry. 40p, Rs.4.50.

Braham Dutt [1972] Deficiency diseases of livestock; symptomology, pathology, daignosis and prevention. 100p. Rs.5.40. (Tech. Bull (AH), 22).

Definition of characteristics of cattle and buffalo breeds in India [1973]. 56p+xvi plates, Rs.6.00 (Bull. ser.14) 3rd Rev. ed.,1979.

Kumar, S. [1976] The African Horse Sickness (34p., Rs.5.00), ICAR Tech. Bull. (A.H.), 15.

Acharaya, R. M., Balain, D. S. and Mani Mohan. [1977] Genetic analysis of a closed herd of Haryana cattle. iv +94p. Rs.9.50.

Chaudhari, R. P. [1977] Bharat men paltu pashupakshiyon ki keetvyadhiyan (Hindi). 68p Rs.3.60.

Singh, S. and Srivastava, H.D. [1977] Diagnosis and treatment of helminthic infections. 96p. Rs.9.50.

Gill, B. S. [1977] Trypanosomes and trypanomsomiasis of Indian livestock. 136p, Rs.30.00. Characteristics of Cattle and Buffalo Breeds [1979] Ed.3 (58p, 17 plates, Rs.6.80). Research in Animal Production [1982] (697p, Rs.47.00)

Adlakha, S. C. [1982] Rinderpest. 61p. Rs. 6.50.

IVRI PUBLICATIONS

The following publications may be obtained from I/C Communication Centre, Indian Veterinary Research Institute, Izatnagar-243 122 (UP).

Bansal, R. P. [1986] Monograph on diagnosis of Rinderpest. (Price Rs.17.00).

Verma Rishendra and Iyer, P.K. R. [1986] Monograph on mycotic infection in animals in India. (Rs.23.00).

Singh, U. B., Dhar, N., Pande, J. K., Singh, L.N., Kumar, A and Mehra, U.R. [1986] Application of nuclear energy in Animal Reproduction and Health Research

Bajpai, K. K. and Sundaram, N. [1986] Handbook on assessment procedure for scientific and technical personnel in ICAR system. (Unpriced).

Bajpai, K. K. and Sundaram, N. [1987] First training programme on office rules and procedures. (Unpriced)

Bajpai, K. K. and Sundaram, N. [1987] Handbook of office (Unpriced).

Bhat, P. N. and Taneja, V. K. [1987] Monograph on genetics and breeding of river buffalo. (Rs.27.00)

Nath, Kedar and Agrawal, D. K. [1987] Urea-Baggasse-molasses: A sustenance feed during scarcity conditions. (Rs. 3.00).

Nath, kedar and Agrawal, D. K. [1987] Water washed neem cake, a cattle feed under scarcity conditions. (Rs.3.00).

Pathak, N. N. [1988] Animal wastes for livestock feeding (Unpriced)

Pathak, N. N. [1988] Nutritional enrichment for livestock feeding. (Unpriced)

Srivastava, A. K. [1988] Biotechnology in Animal Health and Reproduction. (Unpriced).

Handbook of uniforms of Group "C" and "D" employees of ICAR. Published by Communication Centre, IVRI, Izatnagar (Unpriced).

Pathak, N. N. [1990] Gao Avam Vansh Banshi Pasu Prashan Pradishika. (Unpriced).

Somvanshi, R. [1990] 100 years of IVRI Aithihasik Tathya Avam Uplabdhiyan. (Unpriced).

Daniel, S. J. and Hasan, Q. Z. [1990] Fodder production of ruminants. (Unrpiced)

Verma Rishendra and Gupta, B. R. [1990] Monograph on Animal Tuberculosis. [Rs.40.00].

Commemorative volume (Centenary celebrations) [1989-1990], IVRI, Izatnagar. Published by Communication Centre,IVRI, Izatnagar. (Unpriced).

Souvenir 100 years of service to the Nation [1889-1989]. Published by Communication Centre, IVRI, Izatnagar. (Unpriced).

Srivastava, S. K. and Harbola, P.C. [1990] Manual on Procedure for isolation and identification of Leptospira and diagnosis of leptospiroisis. (Rs. 14.00).

Verma, K. C., Panisup, A. S. and Mohanty, G. C. [1990] Monograph on Infectious Bursal disease in Chicken. (Rs. 40.00).

Panisup, A. S., verma, K. C. and Mohanty, G. C. [1993] Manual on avian leukosis sarcoma virus infection. (Rs. 8.00).

Gupta, B. R. and Verma, J. C. [1993] Monograph on Animal Salmonellosis. (Rs. 36.00).

IVRI Organisational set up, Programmes and Activities [1993] Published by Communication Centre, IVRI, Izatnagar. (Unpriced)

Saraswat, M. L. [1993] Eak Bar Kisan Ne Pucha. (Unpriced)

Tripathi, H. and Kunzru, O. N. [1993] Social Research in Animal Sciences, Measurement Techniques. (Unpriced)

Jana, D. N. and Nautiyal, L. P. [1993] Bulletin on Dairy Herd Management. (Rs. 8.00).

Verma, R. P., Mohan, G and Benjamin, B. R. [1994] Bulletin on Crenellation Pattern Technique (CPT). (Rs. 10.00)

Pathak, N. N. [1994] Monograph on introduction to Yak Husbandry. (Rs.26.00).

Kumar Satish [1994] Bovine reproduction a rural experience. (Rs.24.00).

Pathak, N. N. [1996] Nutrition and Feeding of male buffalo

calves for the production of meat (Buffer) and working animals. (Rs.21.00).

Pathak, N. N. [1996] Calf rearing on simple diets evolved at IVRI. (Rs. 17.00).

CARI Publications

Ahuja, S. D. [1994] Layer Cage Management (Rs.6.00)

Panda, B. and Srivastava, A. K. [1996] Bathak Palan (Rs.30.00)

Panda, B. and Mohapatra, S. C. [1989] Poultry Production

Kukut Palan (Hindi) (Rs.20.00)

IAAVR Publications

Verma, Rishendra , Swarup, Devendra and **Jaiswal, T. N.** [1994] *Advances in Veterinary Research and Their Impact on Animal Health and Production.* Published by Indian association for the Advancement of Veterinary Research, 363 Bari Bamanpuri, Bareilly-243 003 (UP).

Chauhan, R. S., Sharma, P. C., Kumar, Rakesh, Sharma, R and **Mahipal, S. K.** [1995] *Advances in Animal Health & Production.* Published by Indian association for the Advancement of Veterinary Research, Bareilly (333 pages).

Verma, Rishendra, Johari, D. C. and **Sharma, Deepak** [1996] *Prospects of Livestock and Pountry Development in 21st Century.* Published by Indian association for the Advancement of Veterinary research, Bareilly. (254 pages).

Verma Rishendra, Singh, S.N. and **Shinghal, K.R.** [1997] *Biotechnology in Animal Health and Production for Economic Development in Asia in Respect of Global Scenario.* Published by Indian Association for the Advancement of Veterinary Research, Bareilly (UP) (182 pages).

Verma Rishendra, Bagherwal, R.K. Nanavati, S. and **Varma, T.K.** [1998] *Advancements in Veterinary Science.* Published by Indian Association for the Advancement of Veterinary Research, Bareilly (U.P.)